Evidence-Based Practice

Guest Editors

ROBERT M. SZABO, MD, MPH
JOY C. MACDERMID, BScPT, PhD

HAND CLINICS

www.hand.theclinics.com

February 2009 • Volume 25 • Number 1

SAUNDERS an imprint of ELSEVIER, Inc.

W.B. SAUNDERS COMPANY
A Division of Elsevier Inc.

1600 John F. Kennedy Blvd. • Suite 1800 • Philadelphia, Pennsylvania 19103

http://www.theclinics.com

HAND CLINICS Volume 25, Number 1
February 2009 ISSN 0749-0712, ISBN-13: 978-1-4377-0482-2, ISBN-10: 1-4377-0482-4

Editor: Debora Dellapena

Hand Clinics (ISSN 0749-0712) is published quarterly by Elsevier Inc., 360 Park Avenue South, New York, NY 10010-1710. Months of publication are February, May, August, and November. Business and Editorial Offices: 1600 John F. Kennedy Blvd., Suite 1800, Philadelphia, PA 19103-2899. Customer Service Office: 11830 Westline Industrial Drive, St. Louis, MO 63146. Periodicals postage paid at New York, NY, and additional mailing offices. Subscription price is $282.00 per year (domestic individuals), $446.00 per year (domestic institutions), $144.00 per year (domestic students/residents), $321.00 per year (Canadian individuals), $510.00 per year (Canadian institutions), $383.00 per year (international individuals), $510.00 per year (international institutions), and $189.00 per year (international and Canadian students/residents). Foreign air speed delivery is included in all *Clinics* subscription prices. All prices are subject to change without notice. **POSTMASTER:** Send address changes to *Hand Clinics*, 11830 Westline Industrial Drive, St. Louis, MO 63146. Customer Service (orders, claims, online, change of address): Elsevier Periodicals Customer Service, 11830 Westline Industrial Drive, St. Louis, MO 63146. Tel: 1-800-654-2452 (U.S. and Canada). Fax: 314-523-5170. E-mail: journalscustomerservice-usa@elsevier.com (for print support); journalsonlinesupport-usa@elsevier.com (for online support).

Reprints. For copies of 100 or more of articles in this publication, please contact the Commercial Reprints Department, Elsevier Inc., 360 Park Avenue South, New York, New York 10010-1710. Tel.: 212-633-3812; Fax: 212-462-1935; E-mail: reprints@elsevier.com.

Hand Clinics is covered in *MEDLINE/PubMed (Index Medicus)*, *Current Contents/Clinical Medicine*, *EMBASE/Excerpta Medica*, and *ISI/BIOMED*.

Printed and bound by CPI Group (UK) Ltd, Croydon, CR0 4YY

Transferred to Digital Print 2011

Contributors

GUEST EDITORS

ROBERT M. SZABO, MD, MPH
Professor of Orthopaedics; and Professor of
Surgery, Division of Plastic Surgery,
Department of Orthopaedic Surgery; and
Chief, Hand and Upper Extremity Service,
University of California, Davis School of
Medicine, Sacramento, California

JOY C. MACDERMID, BScPT, PhD
Co-Director, Hand and Upper Limb Centre
Clinical Research Laboratory, St. Joseph's
Health Centre, London; Associate Professor,
School of Rehabilitation Science, McMaster
University, Institute for Applied Health
Sciences, Hamilton, Ontario, Canada

AUTHORS

MOHIT BHANDARI, MD, MSc, FRCSC
Division of Orthopaedic Surgery, Department
of Surgery, McMaster University, Hamilton
Health Sciences, General Hospital, Hamilton,
Ontario, Canada

KEVIN C. CHUNG, MD, MS
Professor of Surgery, Section of Plastic
Surgery, Department of Surgery, The
University of Michigan Health System, Ann
Arbor, Michigan

CYNTHIA COOPER, MFA, MA, OTR/L, CHT
Clinical Specialist in Hand Therapy,
Scottsdale Healthcare, Scottsdale, Arizona

RYAN M. DEGEN, BSc
Division of Orthopedic Surgery, Michael G.
DeGroote School of Medicine, McMaster
University, Hamilton, Ontario, Canada

BRENT GRAHAM, MD, MSc, FRCSC
Director, University of Toronto, University
Health Network, Hand Program, Toronto,
Ontario, Canada

IAN D. GRAHAM, PhD
Vice President, Knowledge Translation,
Canadian Institutes of Health Research;
Associate Professor, School of Nursing,
University of Ottawa, Ottawa, Ontario,
Canada

RUBY GREWAL, MD, MSc
Assistant Professor and Surgeon, Division
of Orthopedic Surgery, University of Western
Ontario, Hand and Upper Limb Centre, St.
Joseph's Health Care, London, Ontario,
Canada

DANIEL J. HOPPE, BSc
Division of Orthopedic Surgery, Michael G.
DeGroote School of Medicine, McMaster
University, Hamilton, Ontario, Canada

CASEY KNIGHT, MD
Chief Resident, Division of Plastic and
Reconstructive Surgery, Department of
Surgery, McMaster University, St. Joseph's
Healthcare, Hamilton, Ontario, Canada

HANS KREDER, MD
Assistant Professor, Department of Surgery;
and Professor, Division of Orthopaedic
Surgery; and Professor, Orthopaedic Surgery
and Health Policy Evaluation and
Management, University of Toronto; Chief,
Holland Musculoskeletal Program; and Marvin
Tile Chair; and Chief, Division of Orthopaedic
Surgery, Sunnybrook Health Sciences Centre,
Toronto, Ontario, Canada

MARY LAW, PhD
Associate Dean and Professor, School of
Rehabilitation Science, McMaster University,
Hamilton, Ontario, Canada

JOY C. MACDERMID, BScPT, PhD
Co-Director, Hand and Upper Limb Centre
Clinical Research Laboratory, St. Joseph's
Health Centre, London; Associate Professor,
School of Rehabilitation Science, McMaster
University, Institute for Applied Health
Sciences, Hamilton, Ontario, Canada

NORMA J. MACINTYRE, PhD
Assistant Professor, School of Rehabilitation
Science, McMaster University, Hamilton,
Ontario, Canada

RICHARD MARTINOFF, MD
Adjunct Associate Professor, Biomedical
Informatics, Health Professions Division,
College of Osteopathic Medicine, Nova
Southeastern University, Fort Lauderdale,
Florida

LESLIE McKNIGHT, MSc
Research Coordinator, Department of Surgery,
Division of Plastic and Reconstructive Surgery,
McMaster University, St. Joseph's Healthcare,
Hamilton, Ontario, Canada

SUSAN MICHLOVITZ, PhD, PT, CHT
Cayuga Hand Therapy Physical Therapy,
Ithaca; Adjunct Associate Professor,
Rehabilitation Medicine, Columbia University,
New York, New York

BRADLEY A. PETRISOR, MD, MSc, FRCSC
Assistant Professor, Division of Orthopaedic
Surgery, Department of Surgery, McMaster
University, Hamilton Health Sciences,
General Hospital, Hamilton, Ontario,
Canada

HELEN RAZMJOU, MSc, PT, PhD(C)
Research Associate, Holland Orthopaedic
and Arthritic Centre, Sunnybrook Health
Sciences Centre; Women's College Research
Institute, Toronto, Ontario, Canada

DAVID RING, MD, PhD
Medical Director and Director of Research,
Orthopedic Hand and Upper Extremity
Services, Department of Orthopedic Surgery,
Massachusetts General Hospital, Boston,
Massachusetts

JEAN-SÉBASTIEN ROY, PT, PhD(c)
Postdoctoral Fellow, School of Rehabilitation
Science, McMaster University, Hamilton,
Ontario, Canada

MELISSA J. SHAUVER, MPH
Research Associate, Section of Plastic
Surgery, Department of Surgery, The
University of Michigan Health System, Ann
Arbor, Michigan

ROBERT M. SZABO, MD, MPH
Professor of Orthopaedics; and Professor
of Surgery, Division of Plastic Surgery,
Department of Orthopaedic Surgery; and
Chief, Hand and Upper Extremity Service,
University of California, Davis School of
Medicine, Sacramento, California

**ACHILLEAS THOMA, MD, MSc,
FRCSC, FACS**
Director, Surgical Outcomes Research Center
(SOURCE); and Clinical Professor and Head,
Division of Plastic Surgery, Department of
Surgery; and Associate Member, Department
of Clinical Epidemiology and Biostatistics,
McMaster University, St. Joseph's Healthcare,
Hamilton, Ontario, Canada

ANA-MARIA VRANCEANU, PhD
Orthopedic Hand and Upper Extremity
Services, Department of Orthopedic Surgery,
Massachusetts General Hospital, Boston,
Massachusetts

DAVID M. WALTON, MScPT, PhD(c)
Lecturer and Graduate Student, The University
of Western Ontario School of Physical Therapy,
London, Ontario, Canada

Contents

Clinicians need accurate, reliable diagnostic criteria for the conditions they evaluate because this is the basis for rational, effective treatment and the estimation of a meaningful prognosis. Standardizing diagnostic approaches wherever this is feasible can reduce variations in care. The development of diagnostic scales has the potential to meet this goal. The approaches to the development of these scales should follow the same measurement principles used in the development of outcome instruments. The concept of consensus is fundamental to understanding how we make diagnoses and should be thought of as a potentially flexible and fluid idea that can accommodate the discovery of new knowledge in our efforts to accurately diagnose medical conditions.

Diagnosis is a primary activity of hand surgeons and therapists. Diagnostic tests can be used to assist in "ruling in" or "ruling out" a condition to best direct prognosis and treatment. However, the assigning of the diagnostic label is not always obvious. Principles of evidence-based practice may help hand care professionals improve their practice in the diagnosis of their patients. Evidence-based practice can be defined in terms of five steps that serve the structure for decision making and ensure optimum use of clinicians' expertise in the diagnosis.

Prognostic studies are designed to investigate factors that impact the outcome of a disease or its treatment. These factors include, but are not limited to, inherent patient characteristics, the state of the disease, and severity of symptoms. The results of prognostic studies can be used to guide the treatment of patients with similar conditions and overall characteristics. It is the purpose of this paper to provide an outline of how to perform an unbiased appraisal of a prognostic study, allowing the physician to assess the applicability of the results to their patient and thereby assist with decision making in clinical practice.

In the fast evolving world of surgical technology, selecting the best surgical treatment in the absence of sufficient evidence is challenging. With the increasing interest in using less invasive surgeries, arthroscopic rotator cuff repair has become popular. Large randomized controlled studies with rigorous methodology are required to examine the differences between this approach and more traditional methods. Until such studies are complete, clinicians need to appraise the present literature cautiously.

The quality of health care is important to American consumers, and discussion on quality will be a driving force toward improving the delivery of health care in America. Funding agencies are proposing a variety of quality measures, such as centers of excellence, pay-for-participation, and pay-for-performance initiatives, to overhaul the health care delivery system in this country. It is quite uncertain, however, whether these quality initiatives will succeed in curbing the unchecked growth in health care spending in this country, and physicians understandably are concerned about more intrusion into the practice of medicine. This article outlines the genesis of the quality movement and discusses its effect on the surgical community.

Increasing data suggest that the traditional clinician-centered or disease-focused, biomedical approach to illness is less effective than a biopsychosocial, evidence-based, patient-centered approach to illness, particularly for chronic pain conditions. This article distinguishes patient-centered care from more traditional and outdated biomedical decisionmaking models; illustrates the complexity of illness behavior with a patient example; delves into the communication issues raised by this complexity, thereby demonstrating how best evidence can sometimes run counter to biases and intuition; provides a summary of evidence that patient-centered care positively affects outcomes; and explores how the shared decision-making approach along with cultivation of good communication skills can facilitate evidence-based practice.

Evaluation of the outcome of evidence-based practice decisions in individual patients or patient groups is step five in the evidence-based practice approach. Outcome measures are any measures that reflect patient status. Status or outcome measures can be used to detect change over time (eg, treatment effects), to discriminate among clinical groups, or to predict future outcomes (eg, return to work). A variety of reliable and valid physical impairment and disability measures are available to assess treatment outcomes in hand surgery and therapy. Evidence from research studies that includes normative data, standard error of measurement, or comparative scores for important clinical subgroups can be used to set treatment goals, monitor recovery, and compare individual patient outcomes to those reported in the literature. Clinicians tend to rely on impairment measures, such as radiographic measures, grip strength, and range of motion, although self-report measures are known to be equally reliable and more related to global effects, such as return-to-work. The process of selecting and implementing outcome measures is crucial. This process works best when team members are involved and willing to trial new measures. In this way, the team can develop customized outcome assessment procedures that meet their needs for assessing individual patients and providing data for program evaluation.

This article explains the concepts of an economic evaluation relevant to evidence-based hand surgery. Cost-effectiveness analysis in hand surgery is increasingly important as health care resources become scarce in most jurisdictions. Hand surgeons need to incorporate the "manager of health care system" competency in their daily practice. Hand surgery literature may claim that "a novel hand technique" is more cost-effective than a prevailing one; it is important that hand surgeons and other users of clinical research appraise such innovation claims before adopting them in their practices. Clinical researchers can use the methodological principles described here for their cost-effectiveness analysis.

Knowledge translation (KT) is an iterative process that involves knowledge development, synthesis, contextualization, and adaptation, with the expressed purpose of moving the best evidence into practice that results in better health processes and outcomes for patients. Optimization of the process requires engaged interaction between knowledge developers and knowledge users. Knowledge users include consumers, clinicians, and policy makers. KT is highly reliant on understanding when research evidence needs to be moved into practice. Social, personal, policy, and system factors contribute to how and when change in practice can be accomplished. Evidence-based practitioners need to understand a conceptual basis for KT and the evidence indicating which specific KT strategies might help them move best evidence into action in practice. Audit and feedback, knowledge brokering, clinical practice guidelines, professional standards, and "active-learning" continuing education are examples of KT strategies.

Hand Clinics

THE CLINICS ARE NOW AVAILABLE ONLINE!

Access your subscription at:
www.theclinics.com

Preface

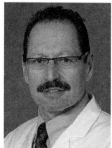
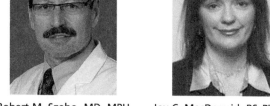

Robert M. Szabo, MD, MPH   Joy C. MacDermid, BScPT, PhD
Guest Editors

Evidence-based medicine is a relatively new concept that rapidly has gained widespread acceptance as an approach to practice and teach medicine. Gordon Guyatt was one of the first people to describe this. In 1990, he described the medical residency at Canada's McMaster University: "Residents are taught to develop an attitude of 'enlightened skepticism' toward the application of diagnostic, therapeutic, and prognostic technologies in their day-to-day management of patients."[1] This approach (which has been called "evidence-based medicine") is based on principles outlined in the book by Sackett and colleagues entitled *Clinical Epidemiology. A Basic Science for Clinical Medicine.*[2] The goal is to be aware of the evidence on which one's practice is based, the soundness of the evidence, and the strength of inference the evidence permits. The strategy employed requires 1) a clear delineation of the relevant question(s), 2) a thorough search of literature relating to the questions, a critical appraisal of the evidence, and its applicability to the clinical situation, and 3) a balanced application of the conclusions to the clinical problem."[1] This issue of *Hand Clinics* is devoted to the increasingly important and relevant application of these principles, which have become known as evidenced-based practice (EBP).

We have assembled a group of outstanding researchers, physicians, and therapists devoted and committed to advancing the practice of EBP, which is the integration of individual clinical expertise with the best available external clinical evidence from systematic research and the integration of patients' values and expectations. EBP is now recognized worldwide as a foundation of quality care, and all surgeons and therapists must embrace the concepts and learn the methods.

To help you become an evidence-based practitioner, this issue will help you develop new skills to find and appraise the best evidence embedded within the volumes of good and bad information available. This issue discusses how to apply these methods to hand surgery and rehabilitation. We must learn how to practice evidence-based medicine. To practice, this issue facilitates the development of new skills by searching literature and internet and provides new skills for the critical appraisal of good and bad information available. In the United States, the Centers for Medicaid and Medicare Services (CMS), health insurers, and certification boards provide the impetus for all of us to put into action EBP. This approach to practice will lead to changes in our behavior.

CMS introduced a "Pay-for-Performance" (P4P) initiative to promote high quality medical care routed in evidence-based medicine by reimbursing toacilitates the development of new skills by searching literature and internet and provides new skills for the critical appraisal of good and bad information available. In the United States, the Centers for Medicaid and Medicare Services (CMS), health insurers, and certification boards provide the impetus for all of us to put into action EBP. This approach to practice will lead to changep performing hospitals at a higher level than poor performing hospitals. Individual health

Hand Clin 25 (2009) xi–xii
doi:10.1016/j.hcl.2008.12.001

care providers are next. The primary objectives of P4P include increasing clinical quality and saving lives. A secondary objective is to improve the cost-effectiveness of health care delivery. Guidelines are becoming more important for insurers who make decisions about authorizing the care of our patients. Government programs like these, with ever increasing practice guidelines, will lead to new expectations in your practice. Whoever controls these initiatives and guidelines, controls medicine, and ultimately, the flow of money. You don't want to be left behind.

Unless individual clinicians and professional associations are sufficiently knowledgeable in EBP to find, disseminate, and implement existing evidence that supports their clinical practices and move towards generating ever increasingly high-quality evidence, health care funders will rationalize removal of payment for services on the basis of insufficient evidence. This is entirely appropriate if high(er) quality evidence supports alternative approaches or if harm is caused. However, funders who do not understand EBP or who wish to hijack the process for their own objectives will have no counterbalance unless individual clinicians and professional associations are adequately informed and competent in EBP. This issue is designed to provide you with the knowledge and skills to start you on your way to practicing evidence-based medicine. We thank all the authors for their hard work, insight, and careful presentation of material in a practical format to achieve this goal.

Robert M. Szabo, MD, MPH
Division of Plastic Surgery
Department of Orthopaedic Surgery
Hand and Upper Extremity Service
University of California, Davis
School of Medicine
4860 Y Street, Suite 3800
Sacramento, CA 95817, USA

Joy C. MacDermid, BScPT, PhD
Hand and Upper Limb Centre Clinical Research
Laboratory
St. Joseph's Health Centre
268 Grosvenor Street
London, Ontario N6A 4L6, Canada

School of Rehabilitation Science, LB33
McMaster University
Institute for Applied Health Sciences
1400 Main Street West, 4th Floor
Hamilton, Ontario L8S 1C7, Canada

E-mail addresses:
rmszabo@ucdavis.edu (R.M. Szabo)
macderj@mcmaster.ca (J.C. MacDermid)

REFERENCES

1. Guyatt G, Rennie D. User's guides to the medical literature: a manual for evidence-based practice. Chicago: American Medical Association; 2002. p. 1–756.
2. Sackett DL, Haynes RB, Tugwell P. Clinical epidemiology. A basic science for clinical medicine. 1st edition. Boston (MA): Little, Brown and Company; 1985. p. xii–370.

An Introduction to Evidence-Based Practice for Hand Surgeons and Therapists

Robert M. Szabo, MD, MPH[a], Joy C. MacDermid, BScPT, PhD[b,c],*

KEYWORDS

- Evidence-based practice • Evidence-based medicine
- Evidence levels • Evidence appraisal
- Outcomes evaluation • Practice guidelines
- Hand surgery • Hand therapy practice

Evidence-based practice (EBP) is a methodical approach to clinical practice where experience, best research evidence, and patient goals and values are integrated to make optimal decisions when making a diagnosis, selecting a diagnostic test, picking an intervention or determining prognosis. There are five steps in this process:

1. Ask a specific clinical question.
2. Find the best evidence to answer the question.
3. Critically appraise the evidence for its validity and usefulness.
4. Integrate appraisal results with clinical expertise and patient values.
5. Evaluate the outcomes

The emergence and evolution of EBP has been associated with an increased quantity and quality of research evidence, a greater need for processes to distil the best evidence, knowledge, and tools to assist with identification and critical appraisal of clinical research evidence, and the emergence of a discipline focused on the translation of knowledge into practice. Hand surgeons and therapists can use the evidence-based process to attain optimal management of individual patients, manage their overall practice, guide the ongoing professional development, and deal with funding and policy makers. Dealing with uncertainty, evidence gaps, and barriers to change in practice can be expected but are manageable, and should lead to redirection of research into areas of importance to practice.

BACKGROUND

Evidence-based medicine (EBM) is now recognized around the world as advancement in the process of providing high quality clinical care. There has been recent focus on the application of this approach in orthopedic surgery[1–3] and hand therapy.[4,5] This issue of *Hand Clinics* is devoted to looking at EBP in terms of its application to hand surgery and rehabilitation.

McMaster University is usually recognized as the birthplace of EBP because of leadership provided by Dr. David Sackett, who led the development of this unique approach while establishing the first clinical epidemiology department at

J.C.M. is supported by a New Investigator Award, Canadian Institutes of Health Research

[a] Department of Orthopaedic Surgery, Hand and Upper Extremity Service, University of California, Davis School of Medicine, 4860 Y Street, Suite 3800, Sacramento, CA 95817, USA

[b] School of Rehabilitation Science, LB33, McMaster University, Institute for Applied Health Sciences, 1400 Main Street West, 4th Floor, Hamilton, Ontario L8S 1C7, Canada

[c] Hand and Upper Limb Centre Clinical Research Laboratory, St. Joseph's Health Centre, 268 Grosvenor Street, London, Ontario, N6A 4L6, Canada

* Corresponding author. School of Rehabilitation Science, LB33, McMaster University, Institute for Applied Health Sciences, Room 429, 1400 Main Street West, 4th Floor, Hamilton, Ontario L8S 1C7, Canada.

E-mail address: macderj@mcmaster.ca (J.C. MacDermid).

Hand Clin 25 (2009) 1–14
doi:10.1016/j.hcl.2008.12.002

McMaster University and contributing to the Oxford Center for Evidence-Based Medicine. Both faculties remain active in teaching others to use and teach EBM and continue to develop these innovative concepts and approaches. However, a variety of like-minded individuals in different countries have also led efforts that have enriched the concepts and sustained their international acceptance. As recognized by David Sackett, the field of clinical epidemiology predated EBM, but provides a significant conceptual basis.[6–8]

EBM as a basis for training physicians developed at McMaster University in Canada in the early 1970s within a new medical school that used innovative "problem-based" methods to train life-long learners who could adapt to rapidly changing information.[9] This training method was shared with other medical faculty and students in Dr. Sackett's landmark and now widely used textbooks.[10,11] The need for adapting practice to new clinical knowledge is even more profound today, with the explosion in availability of scientific journals and other types of information resources. Information learned in medical school will become obsolete and must be replenished with the best new knowledge that will be useful to optimize patient care and outcomes. EBP provides structural and instrumental assistance in making the best possible clinical decisions for specific clinical situations.

DEFINITION OF EVIDENCE-BASED PRACTICE

The one-sentence (first, boldface) definition of EBP has become widely known, but the longer version is more explicit.

Evidence-based medicine is the conscientious, explicit and judicious use of current best evidence in making decisions about the care of individual patients. The practice of evidence-based medicine means integrating individual clinical expertise with the best available external clinical evidence from systematic research. By individual clinical expertise, we mean the proficiency and judgment that individual clinicians acquire through clinical experience and clinical practice. Increased expertise is reflected in many ways, but especially in more effective and efficient diagnosis and in the more thoughtful identification and compassionate use of individual patients' predicaments, rights, and preferences in making clinical decisions about their care. By best available external clinical evidence we mean clinically relevant research, often from the basic sciences of medicine, but especially from patient centered clinical research into the accuracy and precision of diagnostic tests (including the clinical examination), the power of prognostic markers, and the efficacy and safety of therapeutic, rehabilitative, and preventive regimens. External clinical evidence both invalidates previously accepted diagnostic tests and treatments and replaces them with new ones that are more powerful, more accurate, more efficacious, and safer. (From Center for Evidence-Based Medicine, http:// www.cebm.net/ebm_is_isnt.asp and Ref. 7).

THE PROCESS OF EVIDENCE-BASED PRACTICE

Throughout this issue of *Hand Clinics*, the five-step process to EBP will be emphasized to keep this "bird's eye view" in focus, as different authors present examples of how to use the EBP process in different types of clinical decisions or delve into more detail on a specific stage of the process. The authors think this emphasis is worthwhile, as the process itself provides a powerful framework for answering clinical questions, for ongoing personal growth as a clinician, and for better management of health care resources.

The importance of clinical expertise and patient's values in the process is prominent; but neither of these elements are replacements for finding, then evaluating the validity and relevance of clinical research. Rather, these components must be integrated when making clinical decisions. The importance of finding and critically appraising the internal validity or trueness of clinical research before determining its application to the specifics of the individual patients is the defining element of EBP. What follows is discussion of the each of the five steps of EBP listed at the beginning of the article.

Ask a Specific Clinical Question

The first step in EBP is defining the question. Hand surgeons and therapists have many clinical questions that arise from their clinical practice encounters. One of the key elements in EBP is defining specific and answerable clinical questions. The PICO (T) approach is the EBP method for making clinical questions more answerable. This is where clinical experience and knowledge of basic science come into play to help define meaningful questions. Thus, clinical experience is the starting point of EBP. What are the most important aspects of the disease or disability that must be addressed? What are the most important pathologic and prognostic features of the problem? What are realistic outcomes? What are potential long-term risks? These questions indicate how the question posed at the outset of the EBP process reflects clinical experience. The extent to which the question is important to the patient is the beginning of integrating the patient's needs and values.

"P" stands for the important characteristics of the Patient. At this stage, you should choose one to three key features of the patient to make your question more specific. When choosing this, select the most important clinical features. This may be the disease, the person presenting problem, their age, or some key prognostic feature.

"I" refers to the specific Intervention (diagnostic test, prognostic feature, surgical or rehabilitative treatment) that might potentially be used in managing a patient.

"C" refers to the Comparative option (if indicated). This might be a control option (no intervention) or a standard currently accepted therapy.

"O" refers to the Outcomes of interest. This might include specific impairments, such as fracture reduction, hand strength, range of motion, or include activity or participation measures that address concepts like disability or quality-of-life (please see the article by MacDermid and colleagues elsewhere in this issue). This is an area where patient values, goals, and priorities should be embedded within the defined outcomes of interest.

"T" can be added to the acronym to refer to Time. Outcomes are often time-dependent and so the interval of time during which comparisons are made can be an important consideration when determining goals and when comparing across different clinical research studies. This is particularly true in surgical interventions, where postoperative discomforts or complications, short-term recovery, and long-term maintenance of functionality are all important considerations.

Different types of clinical questions can be classified in broad categories. It is important to be familiar with these questions because there are optimal research designs to answers these questions, different threats to validity, and hence different levels of evidence classifications. The following list of topics exemplifies questions asked during different aspects of a clinical encounter (and the categories used in EBP): diagnosis, differential diagnosis or symptom prevalence, prognosis, treatment selection and effectiveness, prevention (diseases/disorders/complications) and harm, etiology, prognosis, and costs (economic and decision analysis).

For example: Your patient is a 45-year-old female who presents with symptoms of carpal tunnel syndrome (CTS). These include numbness and tingling in the radial digits, waking at night, and symptoms that are also brought on by keyboarding. During a pregnancy 5 years prior, she experienced similar symptoms and had pregnancy-related diabetes, both resolved without treatment following the birth of the baby. Upon examination, she has no thenar atrophy, 2-point discrimination is 7 mm, and there is both a positive Tinel's and a positive Phalen's test.

If we consider the patient above, we can ask questions in each of the categories listed.

> Diagnosis: What is the accuracy of a positive Tinel's or Phalen's test in detection of CTS?
>
> Differential diagnosis: In a patient performing repetitive keyboarding with a history of diabetic symptoms, which is more likely to cause numbness and tingling in the hand: radiculopathy, diabetic neuropathy, or CTS?
>
> Symptom prevalence study: What is the rate of concurrent CTS and carpo-metacarpal joint osteoarthritis?
>
> Treatment selection/effectiveness (therapy): Is endoscopic or mini-open carpal tunnel release more likely to resolve symptoms in this patient?
>
> Harm: Which of the above is more likely to result in complications?
>
> Prevention: Would postural retaining or ergonomic computer stations decrease the likelihood of recurrence of musculoskeletal problems when she returns to her job as a keyboarder?
>
> Etiology: Is lumbrical excursion into the carpal tunnel a potential contributor to her nerve compression?
>
> Prognosis: Does a positive Tinel's test (or duration of symptoms) affect the likelihood of success with night splinting for CTS?
>
> Cost-effectiveness: Which is more cost-effective, endoscopic or mini-open release?

Time does not permit us to use point-of-care searches to answer every question for every patient we see.[12] However, if we use the five-step EBP approach to answer patient-specific questions, we can often generalize our analysis to other similar patients. Revisiting recent evidence on these issues will keep us up-to-date in our clinical decision-making. Defining new EBP questions based on our clinical encounters on an ongoing basis will allow us to deepen our understanding of how to manage patients according to best evidence and evolve into more evidence-based practitioners.

Find the Best Evidence to Answer the Question

What we usually rely on as evidence is the opinion that is handed down to us by experts in our fields. There are variations and perceptions with regards to experts. How do we know that their judgments are correct? Surgeons and therapists vary in their perceptions of outcomes of the procedures and treatments. Outcomes should be reported based on clinical evidence. According to expert panels, one-quarter to one-half of the indications for which major procedures are done are inappropriate or equivocal. Experts themselves often disagree on the indications for an intervention or diagnostic test and the effectiveness of different interventions. The practice of medicine has become the art of making adequate decisions based on inadequate information. How many of us have treated our patients with the wrong information provided by "experts" that CTS is caused by using a computer keyboard?

The next step is to search the literature for specific studies or evidence resources that will address our clinical question. The article by Martinoff and Kreder found elsewhere in this issue is dedicated to this process. This is an area where EBP and improvements in technology have supported innovation. The exponential increase in information has been partially offset by increased ways to identify, sort, and evaluate clinical evidence through electronic databases, search engines, and other tools. In fact, there is now research that focuses on optimizing search strategies[13–18] and significant efforts have been invested in providing database access to health professionals.[19,20] Informatics has become a large area of inquiry and development; this discipline focuses on the science of information. It addresses development and analysis of the structure and functionality of natural and artificial systems that store, process, access, and communicate information. The end result is better management of information and increased usability.[21]

It is important to make the process of finding evidence as quick and simple as possible because searching and appraising evidence is consistently reported by physicians and therapists as a barrier to EBP.[22–29] Advancements in finding the best evidence include the development of a whole discipline around evidence synthesis,[30,31] which summarize the best available evidence through systematic reviews (SRs), meta-analysis, and evidence-based clinical-practice guidelines. The Cochrane Collaboration[32–36] has been a leader in the development of these methods in the production and dissemination of SRs.[37] In addition,

DARE (http://www.york.ac.uk/inst/crd/) is a searchable database of SRs that includes a summary and critical appraisal of the SR, so that clinicians can find summaries of the best available evidence on selected topics and review the results of a critical appraisal performed by expert methodologists to assist them with evaluation of the quality of synthesized information.

In as much as finding evidence has been a persistent barrier for clinicians, then a potential solution is to remove the burden of searching and appraising evidence from their hands and put that burden on skilled extractors who classify the evidence as it emerges. This has encouraged the move from "pull-put" to "push-out" of evidence within EBP. A rudimentary form of push-out is when a journal sends out the electronic table of contents of their latest issues to those who sign up for this service. Push-out customized-altering services are a more advanced form of pushing out high quality evidence. Using technology, users can sign up for their clinical interests and receive alerts of evidence pushed out to them based on their needs or clinical interests and preferences for frequency of alerts and quality or relevance cut-offs. Customized user push-out of evidence through alerting services is currently available to hand surgeons through MacPLUS/BMJ Updates (http://bmjupdates.mcmaster.ca/index.asp), although hand surgeons might need to sign-up for both orthopedic surgery and plastic surgery clinical specialties to capture all hand surgery literature. Until recently, this service only covered medical journals, but a MacPLUS Rehab version has been developed and is currently in pilot testing. This should be accessible to hand therapists by 2010. Hand therapists will need to sign up for hand therapy as a specialty and receive alerts about relevant evidence.

Regardless of these advances, there are always clinical questions where primary searching is still required. PubMed is the most commonly used medical database and is freely accessible. A minority of rehabilitation journals are indexed in this database, but the *Journal of Hand Therapy* is included. CINAHL (http://www.ebscohost.com/cinahl/) indexes contains the majority of rehabilitaion journals. The clinician who is not familiar with electronic searching may find this first step a barrier. Fortunately, there are many excellent ways to gain these skills. A variety of written texts and articles are helpful. Pub Med offers excellent online tutorials (http://www.nlm.nih.gov/bsd/disted/pubmed.html). CINAHL offers a free trial. Most university libraries offer (usually free) courses in searching the larger databases. Searching the literature is a skill and, as with most skills, the user becomes more proficient with practice. You will quickly learn that overly broad search terms yield too many articles to review, and will build more efficient searches. Some databases have tools, such as Clinical Queries in MEDLINE, that help you run a more efficient search.

Critically Appraise the Evidence for Its Validity and Usefulness

Critical appraisal

Again, this issue of *Hand Clinics* has an entire article devoted to this step (see the article by Mac-Dermid and colleagues elsewhere in this issue), so the authors will not focus on all the details here. There are recent advances in EBP, which include the proliferation of different critical appraisal tools and critical appraisal services where those proficient in the process perform the critical appraisal.[38] This can make the transition into EBP easier and provides different tools for different study designs or depths of appraisal. The authors caution against abdicating all responsibility for critical appraisal to experts because they do not have the content knowledge of hand surgery and therapy. It is often during the critical appraisal process that clinical logic flaws in the study question or design are revealed. Even one single (critical) design flaw may prevent a study from providing a valid clinical conclusion or may mean that the conclusion does not pertain to the patient of interest. For example, if a case-controlled study was conducted and the CTS patients were population-based, but the controls were those with normal nerve conduction studies recruited from worksites, the estimates of rates and risks for developing CTS would be biased (wrong). Clinical sensibility/external validity and knowledge of research design/internal validity applied simultaneously provide the optimal method for determining if the conclusions presented in a clinical research study should be used as a basis for making a decision about hand surgery or therapy.

There are a number of good references that teach or model the evidence-based process. The classic EBP text written by David Sackett[16] is highly readable and has assisted many clinicians to gain these skills (see http://intl.elsevierhealth.com,/catalogue/title.cfm?ISBN=0443062404 for the sample article on effectiveness).

Law and MacDermid recently published the second edition of *Evidence-Based Rehabilitation*,[39] which provides detailed information/tools within a rehabilitation context. The classic *Journal of the American Medical Association* (JAMA)/*Canadian Medical Association Journal* (CMAJ) series provide

exemplars of the process applied to different clinical scenarios: the article by Roy and Michlovitz elsewhere in this issue follows that model. These exemplars also have accumulated in a textbook format, as have other applications of EBP (http://www.fetchbook.info/Evidence_Based_Medicine.html).

Perhaps the best way for surgeons and therapists to develop these skills is to incorporate EBP appraisal in journal clubs, where both the merits of the research design and the application of the evidence can be discussed with practitioners.[2,40,41] The forms included in this article provide a structured process to evaluate articles that could be used in journal clubs. The Center for Evidence-Based Medicine (http://www.cebm.net/index.asp) provides excellent guidance, forms, and tools to assist with critical appraisal and these are easily accessible online. For those who wish to improve their skills and critical appraisal, the authors recommend a structured critical appraisal form be used to provide more guidance on elements of research design that should be evaluated for different studies. In the article "Critical Appraisal of Research Evidence for Its Validity and Usefulness" by MacDermid and colleagues, they list items from tools and information on how to access a variety of critical appraisal tools. Tools for effectiveness, diagnosis, or outcome measures with the accompanying guide devised by one author (JM) can be obtained by contacting the author or downloading from the website (by permission of author JM). In general, research design principles are designed to evaluate whether a given study can detect true (random sampling and allocation to groups, blinding raters/patients, valid outcome measures), statistically significant (sample size/power, analysis methods), and clinically important (effect sizes) conclusions that will assist in making clinical decisions.

Levels of evidence

One of the primary concepts on rating the quality of evidence that has evolved within EBP is the concept of creating a hierarchy of quality levels based on key elements of study design. By nature, these are gross divisions but have proved to be very useful in increasing awareness of the importance of design quality and in prioritizing and sorting the volume of available information. For example, evidence synthesis may be limited to the highest level of evidence as a means of managing the volume of information and assuring the best evidence is emphasized. While a number of investigators have modified the classic levels system for different applications, the basic concepts remain constant. The most consistently used and most accessible levels rating scale is available on the Center of Evidence-Based Practice Web site (**Table 1**). This hierarchy of evidence classification with which to become familiar considers five levels of evidence, with Level 1 being the highest level of evidence. Level 1 evidence comes from large randomized, clinical trials with clear-cut results and low risk of error, or meta-analyses of randomized trials with homogenous study results and narrow confidence intervals. Level 2 evidence comes from randomized trials with uncertain results or moderate to high risk of error, prospective cohort studies of high quality. Level 3 evidence comes from case-controlled studies or meta-analyses of case-controlled studies. Level 4 evidence comes from case series with no controls. Level 5 evidence comes from expert opinion without critical appraisal, or based on physiology or bench research. The reason randomized controlled trials (RCTs) have been designated as the gold standard is because they are actual experiments where specific questions are discussed by control over variables to minimize selection and information bias, confounding and ruling out chance. RCTs achieve these objectives of design validity, but other research studies can provide worthwhile evidence and should be used where appropriate. EBM is not restricted to randomized trials and meta-analyses, but rather, it involves tracking down the best external evidence with which to answer our clinical questions. It is important to note that there are different optimal designs of different study types. This should be readily observable when examining a level of evidence table where an RCT is the optimal design for individual studies in only one of the five columns (therapy).

For those taking EBP beyond the application to clinical practice into the production of evidence synthesis, then it may be necessary to delve more deeply into the process of making evidence-based recommendations. The most recent developments in this area have been development of guidelines and associated software to assist with this process from the GRADE group.[42–44] In this system, judgments about the strength of a recommendation require consideration of the balance between benefits and harms, the quality of the evidence, translation of the evidence into specific circumstances, and the certainty of the baseline risk. It is also important to consider costs before making a recommendation. This system is more complex than simply using grades of evidence, but reflects the reality that individual pieces of information must be considered within the context of their use.

Determination of relevance

Determination of relevance is the process of deciding whether the findings of internally valid clinical studies can be generalized to your patient. It involves a determination as to whether the results obtained for the specific population (or subgroups reported on) within a clinical research study are similar enough to your patient that you might expect similar results as reported in the study. Matching aspects of the PICO (T) question to the specific demographics (and subgroup analyses) presented within a given trial are critical to evaluating the extent to which evidence can be applied to individual patients.

Integrate Appraisal Results with Clinical Expertise and Patient Values

The point of action is reached when we apply our results to the patient sitting in front of us. Even the developers of EBP have acknowledged that the specifics of how to do this are less clearly defined than are some of the more procedural elements.[45] This issue of *Hand Clinics* devotes an article (see the article by MacDermid and Graham elsewhere in this issue) to the how action requires change in clinical practice behaviors: knowledge translation. But the decision about what specific action should be taken is the point where the clinician must integrate the evidence with the other types of knowledge, including clinical practice experience and patient values. Keep in mind, as Sackett said, "External clinical evidence can inform, but never replace individual clinical expertise. It is this expertise that decides which external evidence applies to the individual patient at all and if so how it should be integrated into a clinical decision."

Sackett[11] termed this "thoughtful identification and compassionate use of individual patients' predicaments, rights, and preferences in making clinical decisions about their care." While some mistakenly assume that EBP conflicts with patient-centered care, in fact, EBP supports it. Hence, this issue has an article devoted to the important issue of client-centeredness and shared decision making (see the article by Vranceanu and colleagues elsewhere in this issue). Not only is this implied in the five steps, but there is evidence suggesting this approach affects outcomes.[46]

Evaluating the Outcomes

The authors fully endorse the importance of evaluating outcomes as the fifth step in EBP. Rigorous evaluation of the treatment outcomes in individual patients is the basis for an ongoing feedback loop that helps you evolve and learn from your clinical experience. It is the difference between "20 years of clinical experience and 1 year of clinical experience repeated 20 times." We are able to better understand the impact of our clinical decisions if we critically evaluate the results of objective tests, performance tests, and patient reports that examine the process and outcomes of our care. In fact, studies confirm that practitioners who experienced improvements in patient outcomes are more likely to continue with evidence-searching.[47] This issue has two articles devoted to this topic, one focused on evaluation of individual patient outcomes (see the article by MacDermid and colleagues elsewhere in this issue), and one that looks at outcome monitoring and its relationship to reimbursement from a broader system level (see the article by Chung and Shauver elsewhere in this issue). Trends in the area of outcome assessment include the development of valid outcome measures specific to upper-extremity disability,[48–53] an entire discipline that focuses on the science of clinical measurement (clinimetrics/psychometrics),[54,55] a greater awareness of the International Classification of Functioning (ICF) as a framework for measuring health outcomes,[56–67] and moves to link reimbursement and outcomes. The move of greater awareness and use of the ICF system has potential advantages for hand surgery and therapy because it recognizes that health extends beyond characteristics of the disease to evaluate how the person functions and experiences life.

CHALLENGES
Misconceptions and Concerns About Evidence-Based Practice

EBP is not without controversy and certainly not without misconception.[68] Debate over these misconceptions and controversies includes clinicians and academics[29] and makes for interesting reading. For example, entries in Wikipedia on EBM have been designated "The neutrality of this section is disputed" (http://en.wikipedia.org/wiki/Evidence-based_medicine) and debates in editorials of scientific journals are common. However, the international spread of the concept is recognized as one of the most substantial changes in conceptual approaches to affect medicine in this century and, thus, is here to stay. Unfortunately, misinformation persists, often from those resistant to learning about EBP or changing their established approach. See the article on knowledge translation by MacDermid and Graham or contact the author (JCM) to learn more about this resistant subgroup.

One misconception is that practitioners are already using evidence as a basis for their practice.

As hand surgeons and therapists, we are constantly being bombarded by new products, new operations, and new methods of treating patients. We are influenced by a technologic imperative. The propensity of health care providers to use technology simply because it is available seems at times to surpass the critical appraisal of its value to our patients. As seen in many of our surgical societies, the most popularly attended courses are skills oriented that present "how to do" a new procedure and often are promoted by industry. In fact, most clinicians do not read, critically appraise, and apply research articles as a means of directing their clinical skills and tend to prefer continuing education courses. Continuing education courses tend to focus on the acquisition of specific skills and place little emphasis on the evidence behind those skills. In fact, the impact of continuing education on the quality of care provided has been questioned.[69] Furthermore, case studies, case series, testimony of experts, and our own clinical experience can create the illusion that an intervention is effective, when in fact a variety of alternative explanations could account for observed changes, including placebo effects, empathy, natural history, and bias.

A second misconception is that EBP takes too much time and that busy clinicians do not have enough time to use these methods. EBP makes clinical practice more efficient, although this is difficult to verify. As with all new clinical skills, there will be some time required to shift approach and a learning curve is expected as these new skills are acquired. Increasingly, the time burden is being lessened by literature synthesis resources and point-of-care decision support aids.

A misconception evident in surgery and rehabilitation is that EBP only values RCTs. A related concern that impacts on surgeon's and therapist's enthusiasm for EBP is the perception that RCTs cannot be well designed and applied in our field because of inherent difficulties in conducting trials in areas where provider characteristics are inherent in the delivery of the intervention. Neither criticism is an accurate representation. While EBP values RCTs, it only requires that clinicians search out and apply the best available evidence. There will always be cases where a weak study or knowledge of anatomy or pathology is the best available evidence. However, this does not mean it is acceptable to continue to rely on these forms of evidence when there is higher quality information that could be used. It is here that we should identify the lack of evidence and direct our research efforts.

Similarly, we acknowledge (and suffer from) the unique challenges in conducting high quality trials in surgery and rehabilitation where the provider

Table 1
Oxford center for evidence-based medicine levels of evidence (May 2001)

Level	Therapy/Prevention, Etiology/Harm	Prognosis	Diagnosis	Differential Diagnosis/Symptom Prevalence Study	Economic and Decision Analyses
1a	SR (with homogeneity[a]) of RCTs	SR (with homogeneity[a]) of inception cohort studies; CDR[b] validated in different populations	SR (with homogeneity[a]) of Level 1 diagnostic studies; CDR[b] with 1b studies from different clinical centers	SR (with homogeneity[a]) of prospective cohort studies	SR (with homogeneity[a]) of Level 1 economic studies
1b	Individual RCT (with narrow CI[c])	Individual inception cohort study with ≥ 80% follow-up; CDR[b] validated in a single population	Validating[j] cohort study with good[h] reference standards; or CDR[b] tested within one clinical center	Prospective cohort study with good follow-up[l]	Analysis based on clinically sensible costs or alternatives; systematic reviews of the evidence; and including multi-way sensitivity analyses
1c	All or none[d]	All or none case-series	Absolute SpPins and SnNouts[g]	All or none case-series	Absolute better-value or worse-value analyses[i]
2a	SR (with homogeneity[a]) of cohort studies	SR (with homogeneity[a]) of either retrospective cohort studies or untreated control groups in RCTs	SR (with homogeneity[a]) of Level >2 diagnostic studies	SR (with homogeneity[a]) of 2b and better studies	SR (with homogeneity[a]) of Level >2 economic studies
2b	Individual cohort study (including low quality RCT; eg, <80% follow-up)	Retrospective cohort study or follow-up of untreated control patients in an RCT; Derivation of CDR[b] or validated on split-sample[f] only	Exploratory[j] cohort study with good[h] reference standards; CDR[b] after derivation, or validated only on split-sample[f] or databases	Retrospective cohort study, or poor follow-up	Analysis based on clinically sensible costs or alternatives; limited reviews of the evidence, or single studies; and including multi-way sensitivity analyses
2c	"Outcomes" research; ecological studies	"Outcomes" research		Ecological studies	Audit or outcomes research
3a	SR (with homogeneity[a]) of case-controlled studies		SR (with homogeneity[a]) of 3b and better studies	SR (with homogeneity[a]) of 3b and better studies	SR (with homogeneity[a]) of 3b and better studies
3b	Individual case-controlled study		Nonconsecutive study; or without consistently applied reference standards	Nonconsecutive cohort study, or very limited population	Analysis based on limited alternatives or costs, poor quality estimates of data, but including sensitivity analyses incorporating clinically sensible variations.

4	Case-series (and poor quality cohort and case-controlled studies[e])	Case-series (and poor quality prognostic cohort studies[k])	Case-control study, poor or non-independent reference standard	Case-series or superseded reference standards	Analysis with no sensitivity analysis
5	Expert opinion without explicit critical appraisal, or based on physiology, bench research or "first principles"	Expert opinion without explicit critical appraisal, or based on physiology, bench research or "first principles"	Expert opinion without explicit critical appraisal, or based on physiology, bench research or "first principles"	Expert opinion without explicit critical appraisal, or based on physiology, bench research or "first principles"	Expert opinion without explicit critical appraisal, or based on economic theory or "first principles"

Abbreviations: CDR, continuing disability reviews; CI, confidence interval; RCT, randomized controlled trial; SR, systematic reviews.

Users can add a minus-sign "−" to denote the level of that fails to provide a conclusive answer because of:

1. EITHER a single result with a wide Confidence Interval (such that, for example, an absolute risk reduction in an RCT is not statistically significant but whose CIs fail to exclude clinically important benefit or harm);
2. OR a systematic review with troublesome (and statistically significant) heterogeneity;

3. Such evidence is inconclusive, and therefore can only generate Grade D (see below) recommendations.

Good, better, bad and worse refer to the comparisons between treatments in terms of their clinical risks and benefits.

Grades of recommendation are as follows:

A: Consistent level 1 studies.

B: Consistent level 2 or 3 studies or extrapolations (where data is used in a situation which has potentially clinically important differences than the original study situation) from level 1 studies.

C: Level 4 studies or extrapolations from level 2 or 3 studies.

D: Level 5 evidence or troublingly inconsistent or inconclusive studies of any level.

[a] {PRIVATE} By homogeneity we mean a SR that is free of worrisome variations (heterogeneity) in the directions and degrees of results between individual studies. Not all SRs with statistically significant heterogeneity need be worrisome, and not all worrisome heterogeneity need be statistically significant. As noted above, studies displaying worrisome heterogeneity should be tagged with a "−" at the end of their designated level.

[b] Clinical decision rule. (These are algorithms or scoring systems, which lead to a prognostic estimation or a diagnostic category.)

[c] See note #2 above for advice on how to understand, rate, and use trials or other studies with wide CIs.

[d] Met when all patients died before the Rx became available, but some now survive on it; or when some patients died before the Rx became available, but none now die on it.

[e] By poor quality cohort study, the authors mean one that failed to clearly define comparison groups or failed to measure exposures and outcomes in the same (preferably blinded), objective way in both exposed and nonexposed individuals or failed to identify or appropriately control known confounders or failed to carry out a sufficiently long and complete follow-up of patients. By poor quality case-control study, the authors mean one that failed to clearly define comparison groups or failed to measure exposures and outcomes in the same (preferably blinded), objective way in both cases and controls or failed to identify or appropriately control known confounders.

[f] Split-sample validation is achieved by collecting all the information in a single tranche, then artificially dividing this into "derivation" and "validation" samples.

[g] An "Absolute SpPin" is a diagnostic finding whose specificity is so high that a positive result rules-in the diagnosis. An "Absolute SnNout" is a diagnostic finding whose sensitivity is so high that a negative result rules-out the diagnosis.

[h] Good reference standards are independent of the test, and applied blindly or objectively to applied to all patients. Poor reference standards are haphazardly applied, but still independent of the test. Use of a nonindependent reference standard (where the test is included in the reference, or where the testing affects the reference) implies a level 4 study.

[i] Better-value treatments are clearly as good but cheaper, or better at the same or reduced cost. Worse-value treatments are as good and more expensive, or worse and the equally or more expensive.

[j] Validating studies test the quality of a specific diagnostic test, based on prior evidence. An exploratory study collects information and trawls the data (eg, using a regression analysis) to find which factors are significant.

[k] By poor quality prognostic cohort study, the authors mean one in which sampling was biased in favor of patients who already had the target outcome, or the measurement of outcomes was accomplished in less than 80% of study patients, or outcomes were determined in an unblinded, nonobjective way, or there was no correction for confounding factors.

[l] Good follow-up in a differential diagnosis study is greater than 80%, with adequate time for alternative diagnoses to emerge (eg, 1 to 6 months acute; 1 to 5 years chronic)

Courtesy of Phillips R, Ball C, Sackett D, et al. November 1998, recent update 2001. Available at: http://www.cebm.net/index.aspx?o=1025. Accessed December 12, 2008; with permission.

and the intervention are linked. Further complicating the challenge is the fact that neither surgery nor rehabilitation is comprised of a single active ingredient (such as a drug) that can be defined or manipulated. Variations between surgical approach, intraoperative techniques and ancillary procedures, postoperative regimen, timing, and content of rehabilitation programs, both individually and in combination, contribute to interventions that are unique and customized to the individual, while also reflecting provider preferences and system influences. Despite the challenges, high quality RCTs are possible and there are design alternatives to help address some of the barriers.

Finally, clinicians are often concerned that the underlying reason for EBP is cutting costs. Hand surgeons and therapists feel at-risk in a competitive health care environment without sufficient high quality evidence to demonstrate the effectiveness of many techniques that they use with confidence. It is important to note that EBP was designed to help identify the most effective treatment, even when that treatment is more expensive. Unfortunately, there are many competing interests in the health care systems and the use of evidence at the system level is a challenge.[26,70] It is possible to abuse the principles of EBP by using the blanket statement "there is no evidence for that" to deny payment for treatment where no RCTs exist. The authors contend that the best defense against this form of abuse is for clinicians and professional associations to have sufficient awareness and activity around EBP that they are able to adequately address any manipulations of the process.

STRATEGIES FOR DEALING WITH EVIDENCE-BASED PRACTICE

The most significant barriers to practicing EBP in hand surgery and therapy practice are: lack of time to find and appraise articles,[23–25,28,29,71,72] lack of skills in critical appraisal,[24,71,73] and lack of Level 1 evidence for many hand surgery and therapy techniques.[74] Each of these barriers presents a real challenge, but there are solutions.

Time is the most consistently reported barrier. A study of the time required to use EBP in surgery indicated that a substantial amount of the time requires searching and retrieving articles.[75] Although EBP should save time by reducing the time spent on ineffective procedures, this is difficult to assess objectively. However, it has been shown that social and cultural factors are better discriminators of high and low evidence use than technical factors,[12] suggesting that those who are committed to using EBP find time less of a barrier.

One of the strategies that can help reduce the time required to search and appraise articles is to use compilations of presynthesized evidence, such as SRs, clinical practice guidelines, and meta-analyses. Another strategy is to use technology support to help keep you informed of emerging evidence. Hand surgery and therapy journals provide e-mail updates of their table of contents, and this can be a very time-efficient way to scan for relevant evidence. If you are affiliated with a university library, the librarian can set up a search that could be rerun and e-mailed to you on a regular basis. This option can be set up manually in PubMed as well. Another option is to use volunteers or students to conduct your searches. Many journals are available online and full access through subscription or online purchase of selected articles can be used to obtain relevant evidence. A good place to develop critical appraisal skills is in journal clubs. Rather than reviewing the latest issue of the *Journal of Hand Surgery* or *Journal of Hand Therapy*, consider reviewing several articles on a specific topic and assign evidence reviews. The American Society of Hand Therapists and the American Society for Surgery of the Hand provide an online journal club for members. A journal club is a useful mechanism for engaging with others to incorporate the clinical application (knowledge translation) into the appraisal process, and thus see immediate relevance and impact on your practice.[39,40,76]

Practice and periodic training or mentorship is needed to improve skills in critical appraisal. The information can be acquired through texts, but asking a local researcher to provide a seminar or two on the topic is probably more time efficient. It is useful to discuss issues, such as bias, controls, follow-up issues, and outcome measures with others. Periodic input from experienced appraisers and researchers can provide a means to speed up the learning curve associated with critical appraisal.

The solution to a lack of RCTs is twofold. First, there is a need for a greater number of RCTs investigating hand surgery and hand therapy interventions. Both professions can (and should) facilitate this through specific opportunities and funding allocated to development of clinical trial expertise and grantsmanship, researcher networking opportunities, and pilot funds that could assist investigative teams in becoming more competitive for more substantial external funding. A second aspect of this issue is that clinicians must be prepared to practice EBP in the face of uncertainty and limitations of less than ideal evidence. Sometimes, bench research or case series evidence is all we have. We can also use our critical appraisal skills to discriminate potential sources of bias among studies characterized as lower levels of evidence. EBP does not mean excluding treatments where only low levels of evidence exist. It does mean that we need to change our practice when more effective treatments have been identified.

THE EVIDENCE-BASED PRACTICE APPROACH WILL CHANGE OUR BEHAVIOR
Initiatives

In the United States, the Centers for Medicaid and Medicare Services (CMS), health insurers, and certification boards are already providing the impetus for all of us to implement EBP. CMS, the largest third-party payer in the United States, has introduced the pay-for-performance initiative. This is a new program designed to promote high quality medical care based on EBM by reimbursing top-performing hospitals at a higher level than poorly performing hospitals. The primary objectives of this program include increasing clinical quality and saving lives. A secondary objective is to improve the cost-effectiveness of health care delivery. It won't be long before the government will reimburse us not for what procedures we do, but for how well we alleviate our patients' maladies.

Other initiatives we are facing include value-based purchasing (VBP) and the Physician Quality Reporting Initiative. The idea of value-based health care purchasing is that buyers should hold providers of health care accountable for both cost and quality of care. VBP weighs information on health care quality, such as patient outcomes and health status, against data on the money spent on health. VPB emphasizes managing the use of the health care system to reduce inappropriate care and to recognize and reward the best-performing providers. VBP refers to any purchasing practices aimed at improving the value of health care services, where value is a function of both quality and cost. VBP requires physicians to demonstrate value by reporting their performance based on quality, efficiency, and patient-experience measures. VBP ties elements of reimbursement to physician's willingness to be held accountable based on such measures and to report to the public on the results. Payers, pushed by purchasers, initially led the movement. The pressure to reduce costs has led to the introduction of performance and efficiency measures as a condition of contracts. Physician-specific performance data is being disclosed to inform consumers and generate evidence-based benefit

design concepts. On July 1, 2007, CMS launched the Physician Quality Reporting Initiative, a voluntary reporting program that encourages quality improvement through the use of clinical performance measures on a variety of clinical conditions. Physicians who successfully report on a designated set of quality measures through claims had the opportunity to earn a bonus payment, subject to a cap, of 1.5% of total allowed charges for covered Medicare physician fee-schedule services. There were 74 measures, with 10 classified under a larger rubric of osteoporosis and perioperative care that may apply to hand or orthopedic surgeons.

Practice Guidelines

Another concern of potential great impact is guidelines. As hand surgeons and therapists, we must develop the tools that external agencies will use to judge us or someone else will do it for us. We should learn from our mistakes. The American College of Occupational and Environmental Medicine (ACOEM) developed workman's compensation treatment guidelines for managed care companies in California. These guidelines are now said to be evidence-based, but because so little good evidence is used, they are no better than expert opinions, and the experts used are not the experts that the authors would expect to write the guidelines for their patients. For example, the ACOEM guidelines state that in all cases of cubital tunnel syndrome, simple decompression alone is the only procedure indicated because workers so treated have fewer days off from work, thus saving the employer money. The authors' experience and evidence both indicate that this is poor advice. Evidence-based guidelines need to be developed to support appropriate therapy for hand patients. MacDermid identified 44 clinical practice guidelines written for hand therapists and found that most were low in quality because of lack of systematic reviews, lack of multidisciplinary teams, inadequate description of the methods of obtaining evidence, the synthesis of recommendations, or the process of external review. Only 2 of the 44 clinical practice guidelines were evidence based. MacDermid concluded: "Practice guidelines published by the American Society of Hand Therapists may be useful in marketing-education, but do little to advance the practice or quality of care." She also stated: "We need to do better. The American Society of Hand Therapists, American Physical Therapy Association, and the American Academy of Orthopaedic Surgery are currently moving toward evidence-based practice guidelines.

Properly developed guidelines involve multiple disciplines, a thorough search and appraisal of the evidence, and a formal process of making recommendations that is linked to the strength of the evidence."[77]

SUMMARY

Evidence-based practice is a methodical approach to using the best available research data to improve clinical decision-making on individual patients or groups. The failure to find good evidence should be a springboard for appropriate research. We can design and participate in multi-center, prospective RCTs. We must make a continuous effort to improve our knowledge using scientific methodology. We need to make the paradigm shift from a traditional practice being opinion-based to a practice involving question formulation, validity assessment of available studies, and appropriate application of research evidence to individual patients. The results will be improved patient outcomes. Different aspects of this process are highlighted in this issue of *Hand Clinics*.

REFERENCES

1. Bhandari M, Zlowodzki M, Cole PA. From eminence-based practice to evidence-based practice: a paradigm shift. Minn Med 2004;87(4):51–4.
2. Dirschl DR, Tornetta P III, Bhandari M. Designing, conducting, and evaluating journal clubs in orthopaedic surgery. Clin Orthop Relat Res 2003;413:146–57.
3. Goldhahn S, Audige L, Helfet DL, et al. Pathways to evidence-based knowledge in orthopaedic surgery: an international survey of AO course participants. Int Orthop 2005;29(1):59–64.
4. MacDermid JC. An introduction to evidence-based practice for hand therapists. J Hand Ther 2004;17(2):105–17.
5. MacDermid JC. (Guest editorial). Evidence-based practice. J Hand Ther 2004;17(2):103–4.
6. Sackett DL. Clinical epidemiology: what, who, and whither. J Clin Epidemiol 2002;55(12):1161–6.
7. Sackett DL. Evidence-based medicine. Semin Perinatol 1997;21(1):3–5.
8. Sackett DL. Clinical epidemiology. Am J Epidemiol 1969;89(2):125–8.
9. Leeder SR, Sackett DL. The medical undergraduate programme at McMaster University: learning epidemiology and biostatistics in an integrated curriculum. 875. Med J Aust 1976;2(23):875, 878–80.
10. Sackett DL, Haynes RB, Tugwell P. Clinical epidemiology. A basic science for clinical medicine. 1st edition. Boston: Little, Brown and Company; 1985.
11. Sackett DL, Straus SE, Richardson WS, et al. Evidence-based medicine. How to practice and teach EBM. 2nd edition. Toronto: Churchill Livingstone; 2000.
12. Gosling AS, Westbrook JI, Coiera EW. Variation in the use of online clinical evidence: a qualitative analysis. Int J Med Inf 2003;69(1):1–16.
13. Haynes RB, Wilczynski N, McKibbon KA, et al. Developing optimal search strategies for detecting clinically sound studies in MEDLINE. J Am Med Inform Assoc 1994;1(6):447–58.
14. Haynes RB, Kastner M, Wilczynski NL. Hedges team. Developing optimal search strategies for detecting clinically sound and relevant causation studies in EMBASE. BMC Med Inform Decis Mak 2005;5(1):5–8.
15. Haynes RB, Wilczynski NL. Optimal search strategies for retrieving scientifically strong studies of diagnosis from Medline: analytical survey. BMJ 2004;328(7447):1040.
16. Montori VM, Wilczynski NL, Morgan D, et al. Optimal search strategies for retrieving systematic reviews from Medline: analytical survey. BMJ 2005;330(7482):68.
17. Wilczynski NL, Haynes RB. Optimal search strategies for detecting clinically sound prognostic studies in EMBASE: an analytic survey. J Am Med Inform Assoc 2005;12(4):481–5.
18. Wong SS, Wilczynski NL, Haynes RB. Developing optimal search strategies for detecting clinically relevant qualitative studies in MEDLINE. Medinfo 2004;2004:311–6.
19. Herbert R, Moseley A, Sherrington C. PEDro: a database of randomised controlled trials in physiotherapy. Health Inf Manag 1998;28(4):186–8.
20. Sherrington C, Herbert RD, Maher CG, et al. PEDro. A database of randomized trials and systematic reviews in physiotherapy. Man Ther 2000;5(4):223–6.
21. Stefanelli M. Knowledge management to support performance-based medicine. Methods Inf Med 2002;41(1):36–43.
22. Bennett S, Tooth L, McKenna K, et al. Perceptions of evidence-based practice: a survey of Australian occupational therapists. Aust Occp Ther J 2003;50(1):13–22.
23. Dysart AM, Tomlin GS. Factors related to evidence-based practice among U.S. occupational therapy clinicians. Am J Occup Ther 2002;56(3):275–84.
24. Jette DU, Bacon K, Batty C, et al. Evidence-based practice: beliefs, attitudes, knowledge, and behaviors of physical therapists. Phys Ther 2003;83(9):786–805.
25. Kamwendo K. What do Swedish physiotherapists feel about research? A survey of perceptions, attitudes, intentions and engagement. Physiother Res Int 2002;7(1):23–34.

26. Laupacis A. The future of evidence-based medicine. Can J Clin Pharmacol 2001;8(Suppl A):6A–9A.

27. Newman M, Papadopoulos I, Sigsworth J. Barriers to evidence-based practice. Intensive Crit Care Nurs 1998;14(5):231–8.

28. Palfreyman S, Tod A, Doyle J. Comparing evidence-based practice of nurses and physiotherapists. Br J Nurs 2003;12(4):246–53.

29. Young JM, Ward JE. Evidence-based medicine in general practice: beliefs and barriers among Australian GPs. J Eval Clin Pract 2001;7(2):201–10.

30. Greenhalgh T. Papers that summarise other papers (systematic reviews and meta-analyses). BMJ 1997;315(7109):672–5.

31. Hatala R, Keitz S, Wyer P, et al. Tips for learners of evidence-based medicine: 4. Assessing heterogeneity of primary studies in systematic reviews and whether to combine their results. CMAJ 2005;172(5):661–5.

32. The Cochrane Centre. Cochrane handbook for systematic reviews of interventions (pamphlet). 1997: Issue 1.

33. Jadad AR, Cook DJ, Jones A, et al. Methodology and reports of systematic reviews and meta-analyses: a comparison of Cochrane reviews with articles published in paper-based journals. JAMA 1998;280(3):278–80.

34. Olsen O, Middleton P, Ezzo J, et al. Quality of Cochrane reviews: assessment of sample from 1998. BMJ 2001;323(7317):829–32.

35. Sackett DL. Cochrane collaboration. BMJ 1994;309(6967):1514–5.

36. Shea B, Moher D, Graham I, et al. A comparison of the quality of Cochrane reviews and systematic reviews published in paper-based journals. Eval Health Prof 2002;25(1):116–29.

37. Sackett DL. The Cochrane collaboration. ACP J Club 1994;120(Suppl 3):A11.

38. Massy-Westropp N, Grimmer K, Bain G. A systematic review of the clinical diagnostic tests for carpal tunnel syndrome. J Hand Surg [Am] 2000;25(1):120–7.

39. Law M, MacDermid JC, editors. Evidence-based rehabilitation: a guide to practice. 2nd edition. Philadelphia: Slack Publishing.; 2008. p. 1–375.

40. Kirchhoff KT, Beck SL. Using the journal club as a component of the research utilization process. Heart Lung 1995;24(3):246–50.

41. Turner P, Mjolne I. Journal provision and the prevalence of journal clubs: a survey of physiotherapy departments in England and Australia. Physiother Res Int 2001;6(3):157–69.

42. Atkins D, Briss PA, Eccles M, et al. Systems for grading the quality of evidence and the strength of recommendations II: pilot study of a new system. BMC Health Serv Res 2005;5(1):25.

43. Atkins D, Eccles M, Flottorp S, et al. Systems for grading the quality of evidence and the strength of recommendations I: critical appraisal of existing approaches The GRADE Working Group. BMC Health Serv Res 2004;4(1):38.

44. Atkins D, Best D, Briss PA, et al. Grading quality of evidence and strength of recommendations. BMJ 2004;328(7454):1490.

45. Guyatt GH, Haynes RB, Jaeschke RZ, et al. Users' Guides to the Medical Literature: XXV. Evidence-based medicine: principles for applying the Users' Guides to patient care. Evidence-Based Medicine Working Group. JAMA 2000;284(10):1290–6.

46. Bahtsevani C, Uden G, Willman A. Outcomes of evidence-based clinical practice guidelines: a systematic review. Int J Technol Assess Health Care 2004;20(4):427–33.

47. Magrabi F, Westbrook JI, Coiera EW. What factors are associated with the integration of evidence retrieval technology into routine general practice settings? Int J Med Inf 2007;76(10):701–9.

48. Beaton DE, Katz JN, Fossel AH, et al. Measuring the whole or the parts? Validity, reliability, and responsiveness of the disabilities of the arm, shoulder and hand outcome measure in different regions of the upper extremity. J Hand Ther 2001;14(2):128–46.

49. Solway S, Beaton DE, McConnell S, et al. The dash outcome measure user's manual. 2nd edition. Toronto: Institute for Work and Health; 2002.

50. MacDermid JC. Development of a scale for patient rating of wrist pain and disability. J Hand Ther 1996;9(2):178–83.

51. MacDermid JC, Turgeon T, Richards RS, et al. Patient rating of wrist pain and disability: a reliable and valid measurement tool. J Orthop Trauma 1998;12(8):577–86.

52. Chung KC, Hamill JB, Walters MR, et al. The Michigan Hand Outcomes Questionnaire (MHQ): assessment of responsiveness to clinical change. Ann Plast Surg 1999;42(6):619–22.

53. Levine DW, Simmons SP, Koris MJ, et al. A self-administered questionnaire for assessment of severity of symptoms and functional status in carpal tunnel syndrome. J Bone Joint Surg Am 1993;75A(11):1585–92.

54. Marx RG, Bombardier C, Hogg-Johnson S, et al. Clinimetric and psychometric strategies for development of a health measurement scale. J Clin Epidemiol 1999;52(2):105–11.

55. Zyzanski SJ, Perloff E. Clinimetrics and psychometrics work hand in hand. Arch Intern Med 1999;159(15):1816–7.

56. Cieza A, Stucki G. Content comparison of health-related quality of life (HRQOL) instruments based on the International Classification of Functioning, Disability and Health (ICF). Qual Life Res 2005;14(5):1225–37.

57. Cieza A, Brockow T, Ewert T, et al. Linking health-status measurements to the International

Classification of Functioning, Disability and Health. J Rehabil Med 2002;34(5):205–10.

58. Cieza A, Stucki G. New approaches to understanding the impact of musculoskeletal conditions. Best Pract Res Clin Rheumatol 2004;18(2):141–54.

59. Cieza A, Stucki G. Understanding functioning, disability, and health in rheumatoid arthritis: the basis for rehabilitation care. Curr Opin Rheumatol 2005;17(2):183–9.

60. Coenen M, Cieza A, Stamm TA, et al. Validation of the International Classification of Functioning, Disability and Health (ICF) Core Set for rheumatoid arthritis from the patient perspective using focus groups. Arthritis Res Ther 2006;8(4):R84.

61. Harris JE, MacDermid JC, Roth J. The International Classification of Functioning as an explanatory model of health after distal radius fracture: A cohort study. Health Qual Life Outcomes 2005;3(1):73.

62. International classification of functioning, disability and health. World Health Organization 2003. Available at: http://www3.who.int/icf/icftemplate.cfm?myurl=homepage.html&mytitle=Home%20Page. Accessed October 30, 2006.

63. Jerosch-Herold C, Leite JC, Song F. A systematic review of outcomes assessed in randomized controlled trials of surgical interventions for carpal tunnel syndrome using the International Classification of Functioning, Disability and Health (ICF) as a reference tool. BMC Musculoskelet Disord 2006;7:96.

64. Jette AM. Toward a common language for function, disability, and health. Phys Ther 2006;86(5):726–34.

65. Kjeken I, Dagfinrud H, Slatkowsky-Christensen B, et al. Activity limitations and participation restrictions in women with hand osteoarthritis: Patients descriptions, and associations between dimensions of functioning. Ann Rheum Dis 2005;64(11):1633–8.

66. Stucki G, Cieza A, Ewert T, et al. Application of the International Classification of Functioning, Disability and Health (ICF) in clinical practice. Disabil Rehabil 2002;24(5):281–2.

67. Stucki G, Ewert T, Cieza A. Value and application of the ICF in rehabilitation medicine. Disabil Rehabil 2003;25(11–12):628–34.

68. Sackett DL, Rosenberg WM, Gray JA, et al. Evidence based medicine: what it is and what it isn't. BMJ 1996;312(7023):71–2.

69. Sibley JC, Sackett DL, Neufeld V, et al. A randomized trial of continuing medical education. N Engl J Med 1982;306(9):511–5.

70. Glenton C, Oxman AD. The use of evidence by health care user organizations. Health Expect 1998;1(1):14–22.

71. Bhandari M, Montori V, Devereaux PJ, et al. Challenges to the practice of evidence-based medicine during residents' surgical training: a qualitative study using grounded theory. Acad Med 2003;78(11):1183–90.

72. Toulkidis V, Donnelly NJ, Ward JE. Engaging Australian physicians in evidence-based medicine: a representative national survey. Intern Med J 2005;35(1):9–17.

73. Maher CG, Sherrington C, Elkins M, et al. Challenges for evidence-based physical therapy: accessing and interpreting high-quality evidence on therapy. Phys Ther 2004;84(7):644–54.

74. Amadio PC, Higgs P, Keith M. Prospective comparative clinical trials in *The Journal of Hand Surgery* (American). J Hand Surg [Am] 1996;21(5):925–9.

75. Krahn J, Sauerland S, Rixen D, et al. Applying evidence-based surgery in daily clinical routine: a feasibility study. Arch Orthop Trauma Surg 2006;126:1–5.

76. Hatala R, Keitz SA, Wilson MC, et al. Beyond journal clubs. Moving toward an integrated evidence-based medicine curriculum. J Gen Intern Med 2006;21(5):538–41.

77. MacDermid JC. The quality of clinical practice guidelines in hand therapy. J Hand Ther 2004;17(2):200–9.

Finding Evidence: Evidence-Based Practice

Richard Martinoff, MD[a],*, Hans Kreder, MD[b,c,d,e]

KEYWORDS

- Literature search • Clinical guideleines
- Evidence-based surgical practice

Best practice treatment decisions require the integration of external information, internal information, and patient factors. External information is obtained by accessing the best available evidence from the literature concerning the clinical situation at hand. Internal information includes consideration of such local factors as the surgeon's personal experience and skills, knowledge of the available equipment, and support personnel. Finally and perhaps most importantly, inclusion of the patient's preferences in a collaborative model is essential, because different patients assign unique priorities to complications and outcomes. Numerous examples of the heterogeneity of patient perspectives are available in the literature. One that stands out is the case of prostate cancer patients who were given the choice of an operation that would have a higher chance of being curative at the expense of a higher risk of impotence and incontinence. Patients differed in their preferences: some were adamant about undergoing surgery to improve survival, whereas others would rather die sooner but retain continence and potence.[1]

The concepts of evidence-based medicine (EBM) have become ubiquitous in the last decade, permeating all aspects of clinical medicine and producing a torrent of evidence-based guidelines and resources to find research-supported guidance for patient care. The practice of EBM requires a clear understanding of the clinical question being asked by the clinician.[2] This is followed by a competent search strategy against comprehensive online databases of literature and a critical evaluation of the relevance to the particular clinical setting within which the surgeon operates. The conclusions are then applied to provide better care to the patient.[3] This EBM evidence cycle incorporates the formulation of a clinical question into an effective search strategy against literature and guideline databases discussed in this article as the first two steps of the evidence cycle (**Fig. 1**).

Aspects of EBM have increasingly become integrated into operative orthopedic practice. The Users' Guide to the Orthopedic Literature, which has appeared in the *Journal of Bone and Joint Surgery*, enables the practicing hand surgeon to critically evaluate and apply the findings of systematic research. Several specialized sources exist for the aggregation of studies, meta-analyses, and evidence-based guidelines for hand surgery practice. Members of the McMaster University Surgical Outcomes and Resource Center have also published a series of articles, each focused around a surgical clinical scenario, and familiarizing the surgeon with the techniques of EBM in the areas of therapeutics evaluation, diagnosis, literature retrieval, systematic reviews, and self-

[a] Biomedical Informatics, Health Professions Division, College of Osteopathic Medicine, Nova Southeastern University, 3200 South University Drive, Fort Lauderdale, FL 33328, USA
[b] Department of Surgery, Division of Orthopaedic Surgery, University of Toronto, Toronto, Ontario, Canada
[c] Orthopaedic Surgery and Health Policy Evaluation and Management, University of Toronto, Toronto, Ontario, Canada
[d] Holland Musculoskeletal Program, Sunnybrook Health Sciences Centre, Toronto, Ontario, Canada
[e] Division of Orthopaedic Surgery, Sunnybrook Health Sciences Centre, MG 365, 2075 Bayview Avenue, Toronto, Ontario M4N 3M5, Canada
* Corresponding author.
E-mail address: martinof@nova.edu (R. Martinoff).

Hand Clin 25 (2009) 15–27
doi:10.1016/j.hcl.2008.09.002

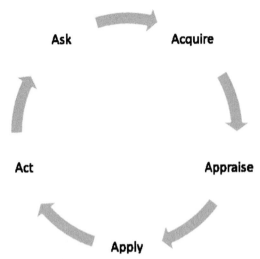

Ask

Acquire

Act

Appraise

Apply

Fig. 1. The evidence cycle. (*Adapted from* Giannoudis P, Bhandari M. Evidence-based medicine: what it is and what it is not. Injury 2006;37:302–6; with permission.)

auytitng.[4] EBM techniques have led to several major shifts in routine practice of hand surgery. One of the foremost examples is the cessation of the practice of giving routine perioperative antibiotics for carpal-tunnel surgery.[5]

Finding the best evidence requires technical skills and awareness of optimal research designs for different clinical questions. Evidence on which to base clinical decisions is not limited to randomized controlled trials (RCT) as the exclusive type of evidence. This research design is impractical for many issues in the field of hand surgery. For example, customization of surgical and rehabilitation techniques to individual patient needs, unique presentations of trauma, rare or unusual disorders, and complexities of handling surgical preferences and expertise are all significant barriers to the conduct of randomized trials. This may account for why randomized trials comprise less than 14% of the published literature.[3] In addition, because hand surgery is a highly specialized field, it is sometimes difficult to gather sufficient numbers of surgeons and cases for a fully powered randomized trial, particularly where clinical problems have a low incidence or prevalence in the general population. This is not to discount the substantial progress made in research addressing these problems, because national and international collaborations allow sufficiently powered studies of low-incidence issues with a large number of patients in such fields as orthopedic trauma.

Observational studies become an important source of shared knowledge in the diagnosis and management of hand problems among the world community of hand surgery specialists. For this reason, surgeons must have the ability to define answerable clinical questions and then identify and appraise high research evidence obtained within literature syntheses, randomized trials, and observational studies to assist in making evidence-based clinical decisions.

This article provides a tested methodology for formulating a structured question from a clinical dilemma and then transforming that question into a query appropriate for searching online evidence-based resources. Also listed are some of the preeminent online databases for searching for evidence pertinent to clinicians specializing in hand surgery. Discussed are various online methods for continuously delivering pertinent evidence to the clinician as it becomes available. The conclusion is a practical example of a literature search as it applies to a problem commonly encountered in surgical care of the upper extremity.

EVIDENCE-BASED PRACTICE AND LITERATURE SEARCH: FORMULATING THE QUESTION

EBM does not discount the value of clinician experience or the uniqueness of each clinical situation. It does promote the integration of clinical expertise with the best external published evidence available. This is best accomplished through a standardized, step-wise process.

The first step is formulating the clinical question to be answered. The different types of clinical questions include those of etiology, diagnosis, prognosis, and treatment. For questions of treatment (A versus B) the best external evidence is contained in high-quality RCTs or in a summary of such studies in a meta-analysis or practice guideline.

The question should be phrased in a clear and concise matter. The population, intervention, comparison, and outcome methodology of formulating a question from a clinical scenario involves constructing a search phrase based on four criteria: (1) the population of interest, (2) the intervention contemplated, (3) the alternative courses of action, and (4) the outcome of interest (**Table 1**).[6,7] This is an essential step in facilitating future searches and is not often as easy as it seems.[8] The formulated question now contains keywords that become the search terms for the online search. Imprecise or general keywords lead to a large number of retrieved references, many of which are not pertinent. Although the speed of retrieval of online searches is no longer a concern, the clinician has to devote significant time and effort to reviewing the search results and discarding a significant portion of them because of irrelevance (**Table 1**).

Table 1
The population, intervention, comparison, outcome method

Step	Description
Population	For patients with lateral epicondyliti...
Intervention	Will corticosteroid injection...
Comparison	As compared with conservative management...
Outcome	Result in shorter duration of pain?

Data from Birch DW, Eady A, Robertson D, et al. Users' guide to the surgical literature: how to perform a literature search. Can J Surg 2003;46(2):136–41.

After the question has been formulated, the next step is to "distill" that question into a usable search query. It is the keywords in the search query that are compared against the database by the search algorithm. Most search algorithms filter the search query to remove stop words, such as "and," "for," and "with," which are frequently used words that do not add to the relevance of the search. The Medline "negative dictionary" contains a list of such stop words that can be removed from the clinical question by the user.[9] Most search algorithms then use one of two retrieval methodologies; exact-match or partial-match retrieval.[10] Exact-match retrieval algorithms, used commonly in bibliographic databases, use the Boolean operators "AND," "OR," and "NOT" to retrieve a set of relevant articles. Some systems allow the use of wild-card characters, usually an asterisk, so that in the example the keyword "inject" retrieves articles with the terms "inject," "injection," "injectable," and so forth. Partial-match retrieval algorithms, used more often in full-text retrieval systems, produce a relevance-ranking, prioritizing documents by how closely they fit the query.[10]

Various forms of evidence are indexed in databases, such as MEDLINE, either manually by human operators or automatically. The indexing occurs using a controlled terminology, which contains a list of terms representing concepts and the relationships between these terms. The MeSH terminology is used for indexing the MEDLINE databases. Retrieval of relevant documents is facilitated by MeSH subheadings that qualify subject headings into more specific terms. The relationships encoded in the MeSH terminology allow retrieval of articles by terms related to the search term. For example, "lateral epicondylitis" also retrieves articles indexed under "tennis elbow."

The next step is to decide which online tool or database to use for the literature search. The choice of tool depends on user preference, evidence type, availability of the database, and specialization of the database. The starting point for most searches is PubMed, which is an Internet portal for searching the MEDLINE database from the US National Library of Medicine. MEDLINE contains more than 10 million citations from 4000 journals published in the United States and internationally.

PERFORMING A SEARCH IN PUBMED

PubMed may be searched through the National Center for Biotechnology Information by going to http://www.ncbi.nlm.nih.gov/sites/entrez/ from any standard World Wide Web browser. Select "PubMed" from the list of databases to search, and then enter the search terms in the text box. The "MEDLINEPlus" option is often selected as the display type; however, selecting "Abstract-Plus" shows a link to the online, full-text version of the publication, if available. By clicking on the "limits" tab, one can also limit the search to certain authors, journals, publication date windows, age and gender of the studied population, types of articles, and other search delimiters. For example, hand surgeons may find limiting the search results to those with links to full text of the article, published in the last 10 years, performed on humans, published in the English language, and of the RCT type, to be helpful. The default filter may be set to "Review," which produces a listing of results from the query, further limited to review article types. The settings of the search filter can be changed by clicking on the "tools" icon. PubMed automatically combines the text terms for the search using the Boolean "AND" operator, so that all of the terms in the search have to be found in each record retrieved. This produces a more narrowly focused list of retrieved references. An alternate way of searching PubMed is to use MeSH terms. Each reference in MEDLINE is indexed using MeSH terms, and using them in a search may produce a more focused and relevant list of references compared with using solely text search terms. Most hand surgeons are unfamiliar with using the MeSH ontology, and the time and effort involved in learning it may not be worthwhile. For those clinicians who are interested in exploring the MeSH ontology, the National Center for Biotechnology Information MeSH Browser is a useful first step.

To illustrate the impact of search terms, the authors have performed a search on the topic of "Duputyren's contracture" using several search strategies. The first of these was an unqualified search of the term on the popular Google search engine. Because the search engine uses the PageRank algorithm, which lists the various Web pages by popularity, the results are numerous but do not incorporate level of evidence or scientific rigor in the ranking. The Google search produces 83,700 listings, many of which are consumer or patient-oriented Web sites of dubious editorial quality. The authors then performed a search on PubMed of all "Duputryen's contracture" publications, which resulted in 1880 citations. Filtering these results to only those of the "review" type whittled this number further to 144 citations. Further limiting the search to only those trials meeting criteria for RCT brought the number to just 17. No clinical guidelines issued by a specialty professional organization or board were found. This underscores the frequent difficulty of obtaining guidance from literature sources in the field of hand surgery (**Fig. 2**; **Table 2**).

SEARCHING FOR EVIDENCE-BASED MEDICINE BY APPLYING EVIDENCE-BASED MEDICINE FILTERS

Specific clinical queries are available within PubMed at the "PubMed Clinical Queries" page located at http://www.ncbi.nlm.nih.gov/entrez/query/static/clinical.shtml. Three specialized searches are available. These searches represent the use of preformatted methodologic search filters composed of a Boolean combination of search terms by keyword and MeSH subheading when appropriate, such that results of a user query are further focused on a clinically relevant subtype. Adjustments for a narrow and more specific, or broad and more sensitive query can also be made on the search page based on user preference. The first of

these is a "search by clinical study category." This search can further focus results to studies dealing with the etiology, diagnosis, therapy, prognosis of a disease, or clinical prediction guides for that disease.[11] The other clinical query types available are specific to systematic reviews and to medical genetics publications. The specificity and sensitivity of these methodologic search filters are available at http://www.ncbi.nlm.nih.gov/entrez/query/static/clinicaltable.html (**Fig. 3**).

USING PREFILTERED, CRITICALLY APPRAISED WEB SITES

Multiple professional societies for hand surgery exist and may be a valuable source of continuing medical education material and evidence-based practice for the practicing hand surgeon. These include the American Society for Surgery of the Hand, American Association for Hand Surgery, the Hand Rehabilitation Foundation, and the American Academy of Orthopedic Surgeons. Through continuing medical education offerings, annual symposia, and education meetings, these professional societies provide multiple opportunities for updating clinical knowledge. The American Academy of Orthopedic Surgeons and the American Society for Surgery of the Hand are collaborating on developing evidence-based guidelines for clinical practice. The first of these is the guideline on the clinical diagnosis of carpal tunnel syndrome.[12]

Although MEDLINE provides a broad search against the available medical literature, some experts have advocated beginning the search at a preappraised literature review site. In this type

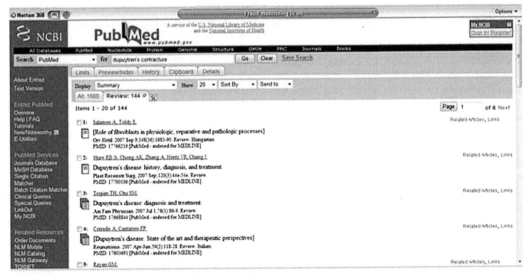

Fig. 2. MEDLINE database search results from PubMed.

Table 2
Search results from various search engines for "Dupuytren's contracture"

Type of Search	Number of Citations
Google "Dupuytren's contracture"	83,700
PubMed "Dupuytren's contracture" (all)	1880
PubMed "Dupuytren's contracture" (review filter)	144
PubMed "Dupuytren's contracture" (randomized controlled trials)	17
PubMed "Dupuytren's contracture" (guidelines)	0
National Guideline Clearinghouse "Dupuytren's"	1

of site, the literature has been reviewed and publications selected based on quality criteria. The Cochrane Library and ACP Journal Club Plus are examples of such sites.

American College of Physicians Journal Club

ACP Journal Club Plus is an online searchable database that is a collaboration between the American College of Physicians and McMaster University. Citations from more than 130 journals are rated for quality by a staff panel, and then rated for clinical relevance by an international panel of physicians. The results of a search on these preappraised literature review sites are usually more manageable than those on MEDLINE. Often the question of interest to the hand surgeon is not answered by a literature-review site, however, and a search against MEDLINE still needs to be performed.

The ACP Journal Club Web site (http://www.acpjc.org/) provides an online search feature for its database of original articles that have been evaluated and summarized in a structured form, with the addition of commentary. The database includes articles of import to practicing internists, and as a consequence most of the included content relevant to hand surgery addresses nonsurgical management of hand problems, interventional techniques that may be performed by internists in the office, and comparison of conservative versus surgical management approaches to problems of the hand. The search may be performed by typing the search terms into the search window on the page available at http://www.acpjc.org/fcgi/imsearch.pl. On this page, one can also select the article type to search for, including "therapeutics," "diagnosis," and "prognosis." Boolean searches can be performed in the search window, such that the search [('myocardial infarction' or 'heart attack') and aspirin] retrieves articles including either the first or second term but always including the third term. Words that are not enclosed in quotation marks in a query are passed through a custom thesaurus, allowing articles with related terms to be included in the search

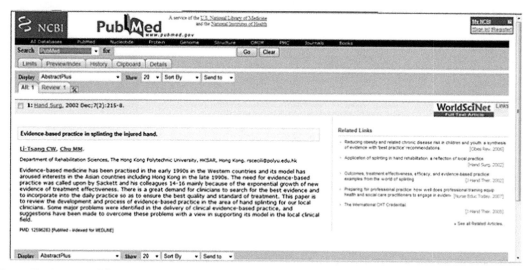

Fig. 3. Citation record from PubMed, with link to full-text article.

results. This thesaurus option can be turned off by clicking the "don't use synonyms" box. Click on the "go" button to initiate the query.

A sample search for "lateral epicondylitis" retrieved five results. All retrieved results contain a link to the PubMed citation and abstract, and the PubMed ID number. These retrieved results often contain star rankings, which are averaged ratings of the article's relevance to practicing clinicians based on the McMaster Online Rating of Evidence system. Articles whose findings are deemed to have high relevance to practicing physicians are then converted to structured summaries, which are available online by selecting the citation. These structured summaries include what question the article is attempting to answer, the design and setting of the article "methods," the "results" and "conclusion," and summarizing graphics if available, and commentary from a domain-expert familiar with the article.

Cochrane Reviews

The Cochrane Library database is a product of the Cochrane Collaboration, a not-for-profit organization, and includes high-quality evidence on the effectiveness and aptness of various therapeutic interventions. The Cochrane Reviews includes reviews of clinically relevant evidence, using methodic search strategies to search MEDLINE, CINAHL, and other online databases. The studies are then included or excluded based on predetermined criteria agreed to by the Cochrane Musculoskeletal Group, and a pooled data analysis using weighted mean differences or a similar statistical methodology is then performed. The Cochrane Reviews incorporates the Cochrane Central Register of Controlled Trials, a comprehensive database of randomized clinical trials in orthopedics and hand surgery. The Cochrane Reviews are published online and in print as the *Cochrane Database of Systematic Reviews*.

A search for "lateral epicondylitis" in the Cochrane Library Web site produced 5 *Cochrane Reviews*, 87 clinical trials, 7 technology assessments, and 1 economic evaluation. The *Cochrane Reviews* retrieved included reviews of the use of orthotic devices, shockwave therapy, and deep transverse massage as treatment modalities, and protocols for reviews of physical therapy modalities and corticosteroid injections in the treatment of lateral epicondylitis (**Fig. 4**).[13]

National Guideline Clearinghouse

The National Guideline Clearinghouse (NGC) (www.guideline.gov) is an initiative of the Agency for Healthcare Research and Quality. It maintains a comprehensive database of evidence-based clinical guidelines from various sources, such as professional organizations and governmental bodies. This database includes structured summaries of the guideline's content and recommendations. It also contains links to the full-text guideline and several tools for working with guidelines, such as a guideline comparison tables (guideline synthesis) and expert commentary.

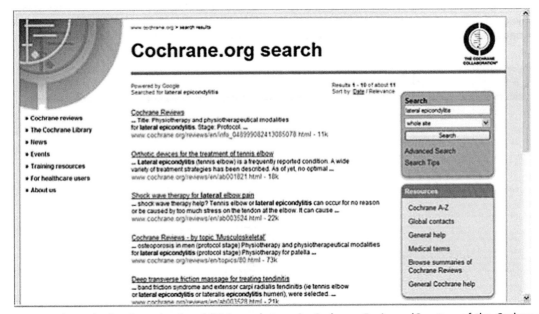

Fig. 4. Search results for "lateral epicondylitis" search term in Cochrane Reviews. (*Courtesy of* the Cochrane Collaboration; with permission.)

A text-input box is available for text keyword searches, and further qualification of search results may be performed by clicking on the "detailed search" link. Searches may be performed in the basic search or detailed search modes. In basic search mode, the NGC search engine searches the contents of the guideline summaries in its database. In detailed search mode, searches are made within selected fields of the database. This allows the user to qualify search results by guideline type, intended users, clinical specialty, evidence evaluation methods, and year of publication. Query terms may be specified using quotation marks for exact searches and Boolean operators. The NGC search engine does attempt to map query terms using a UMLS thesaurus and automatically populates the disease/condition or treatment/intervention fields if matches are found. The NGC search engine also attempts to find the query term as an exact match within the text of the NGC summary of a guideline.

When searching for the term "lateral epicondylitis" in basic search mode in the NGC database, the authors were able to retrieve four results. Although none of the retrieved guidelines addressed lateral epicondylitis exclusively, several interesting results were retrieved. The first of these was a guideline from the American College of Radiology and its Expert Panel on Musculoskeletal Imaging regarding appropriate diagnostic imaging modalities for evaluation of chronic elbow pain. The second of these was a guideline from the American College of Occupational and Environmental Medicine on recommendations for assessing and treating patients with elbow disorders, including recommended ergonomics evaluation and diagnostic and treatment modalities. The search also included a disability guideline from the Work Loss Data Institute covering initial assessment modalities, treatment modalities, and secondary assessment. This guideline also includes the Official Disability Guidelines' Return-To-Work Pathway for lateral epicondylitis. The last of the retrieved guidelines came from the Council of Acupuncture and Oriental Medicine Associates and covered the duration and frequency of acupuncture and electroacupuncture modalities for the treatment of lateral epicondylitis (**Fig. 5**).

Cumulative Index to Nursing and Allied Health Literature

An additional resource for literature search is the Cumulative Index to Nursing and Allied Health Literature (CINAHL). CINAHL includes citations of journal articles, books, chapters, and computer software programs. CINAHL uses a controlled vocabulary called the "CINAHL Headings."[14] One of the advantages of CINAHL is that its database does include the bibliographic references at the end of its articles. The CINAHL database can be accessed directly or through one of the secondary vendors, such as EBSCO or OVID Technologies, available at most institutional online libraries. CINAHL uses major heading key words to limit searches to the article's focus. It allows search by author name and institutional affiliation. Searches may be performed as a simple keyword search or through an expandable tree view using the CINAHL Headings. A simple keyword search for "lateral epicondylitis" on the CINAHL through EBSCO host (a secondary portal for accessing the CINAHL database and integrating it with local online library resources) produced 174 citations. Additional keyword terms are suggested on the left-sided panel of the Web page, and may be helpful for narrowing the search. A search for the term "lateral epicondylitis" using CINAHL Headings produces "tennis elbow" as a suggested major concept, but also numerous unrelated or nonuseful terms, such as "iliotibial band friction syndrome" and "periodontal cyst." Clicking on the relevant term expands a tree view of related "child-nodes" of tennis elbow. Additional subheadings are shown on the right side of the page, one of which is "surgery." One can select the surgery option, and then select "AND" as the Boolean operator in the "combine selections with" selector. This search resulted in 39 citations that have both "tennis elbow" and "surgery" as major headings. This search can be narrowed even further by clicking on one of the suggested subjects now displayed on the screen.

CINAHL also includes the number of times the paper has been cited by other published articles. Quality of systematic reviews, in terms of methodologic rigor and sound statistical analysis, has been shown to correlate with the mean number of citations in subsequent publications in the orthopedics field.[15] When available within a bibliographic index, a publication's number of citations may reflect quality of the study.

PEDro

PEDro is an online collection of publications and guidelines related to evidence-based physiotherapy and rated for quality. PEDro is an initiative of The Centre of Evidence-Based Physiotherapy at the University of Sydney. Trials and guidelines are culled from a variety of resources, including MEDLINE, NGC, prospective searches of literature databases using automated (SDI) optimized searches, and incorporation of the rehabilitation

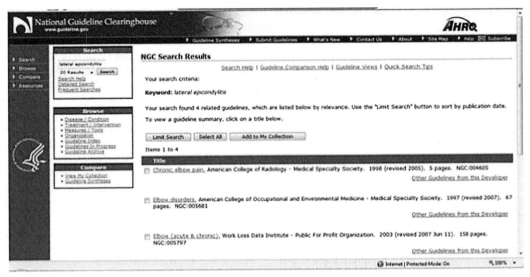

Fig. 5. Sample search for guidelines on the National Guideline Clearinghouse Website.

and related therapies field of the Cochrane Collaboration. The Centre of Evidence-Based Physiotherapy has codified criteria for inclusion of clinical trials, systematic reviews, and practice guidelines. Included trials are then rated on a checklist (the PEDro scale), which rates trials based on internal validity and statistical quality. This is in contrast to the ACP Journal Club site and several other compendiums, which use the Jadad scale for rating study quality. Most of the checklist criteria of the PEDro scale are based on the Delphi list, a list of characteristics thought to determine the statistical quality of a study. The validity of the PEDro scale for rating physiotherapy study quality has been published.[16] Use of the PEDro scale and the Jadad scale for rating quality of RCTs, at least in the specialized literature of stroke rehabilitation, has also been compared.[17]

The PEDro database is updated on a monthly basis. It can be searched by browsing the search page at http://fmweb01.ucc.usyd.edu.au/pedro/FMPro?-db=Sessions.fp5&-format=search_new.htm&-new. Both a simple search and advanced search modalities are available. In the advanced search mode, up to 11 criteria, including abstract and title of the article and the modality of therapy addressed in the publication (ie, strength training) can be searched. Not all of these criteria need to be selected, and selecting three is usually sufficient. Boolean operators can be applied to the search criteria. A query of "lateral epicondylitis" in the abstract and title field and "practice guideline" produced no results. A query of "lateral epicondylitis" in the abstract and title field and "systematic review" produced 15 results. A query of "lateral

epicondylitis" in the abstract and title field and "clinical trial" produced 50 results (**Fig. 6**).

ADDITIONAL RESOURCES

In addition to these unique search sites, the clinician may choose to search within a specific journal's or professional organization's Web site. Such sites as the British Medical Journal (bmj.com) or American Academy of Family Practice (aafp.com) may provide a familiar format and trusted resource for the practicing clinician. Although most of the publications in these periodicals are indexed within PubMed and search portals already mentioned, clinicians may benefit from their value-added resources, such as patient information handouts, and supplementary materials, such as guideline illustrations. For example, a search for "lateral epicondylitis" at the American Academy of Family Practice Web site leads to patient handouts on "tennis elbow" and "exercises for tennis elbow" published in the Academy's publication, *American Family Physician*.[18] Many of these primary resources are available by subscription only through their publishers, although more and more are becoming freely available within a certain time frame after their original print publication.

BMJ Clinical Evidence (http://clinicalevidence.bmj.com) is another decision support resource, with reviews of common clinical conditions and their treatments. The Web site has a search feature against a database of reviews, summarizing evidence from RCTs, observational studies, and guidelines. It provides rankings of helpfulness of

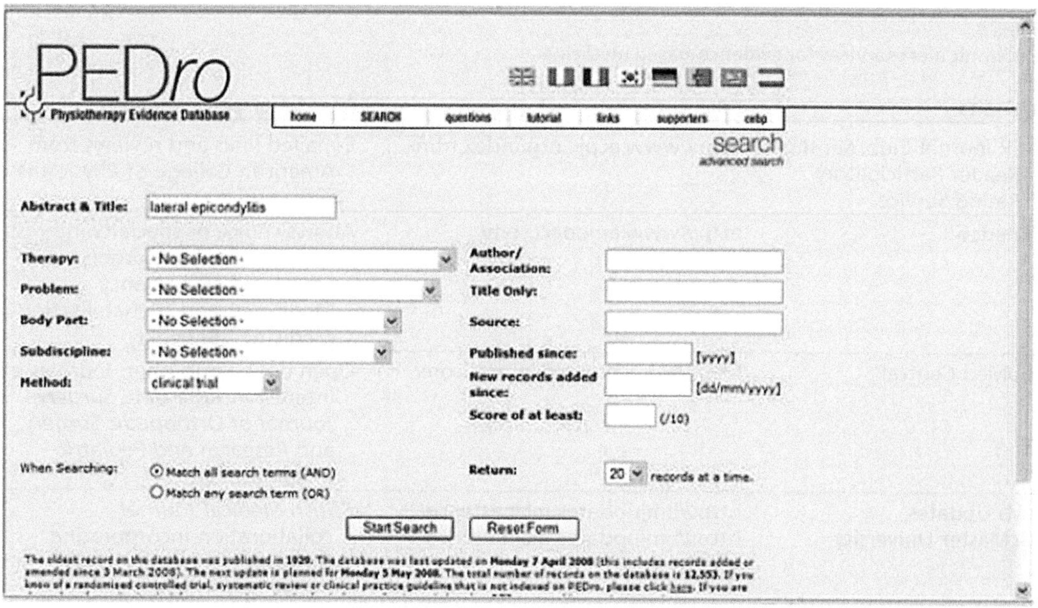

Fig. 6. PEDro database search page. (*Courtesy of* PEDro; with permission. Available at: www.Pedro.org.au.)

various therapeutic interventions, phrased as answers to clinical questions, and links to pertinent publications. Really simple syndication feeds and e-mail alerts of updated material are also available. It is ideal for researching evidence supporting use of one treatment versus another, especially in conditions with a variety of conservative treatments before initiating surgical treatments.

The TRIP database (http://www.tripdatabase.com) was founded in 1997 with the goal of providing evidence-based answers to clinical questions in a clinically relevant time frame. A specialist site for orthopedics is available, narrowing its search to around 20 relevant journals in the field through MEDLINE.

The UpToDate Web site (http://www.uptodateonline.com) is an EBM resource founded by Harvard Medical School faculty and a community of expert authors and editors, integrating evidence-based resources. Its information is geared toward primary care practitioners and non-operative specialties but includes evidence for or against surgical modalities. Information is presented in a narrative format with citation links to original research. In 2006, UpToDate began using UTD-GRADE grading of recommendations, using numbers 1 to 2 for recommendations, and letters A to C for quality of evidence supporting that recommendation.

PUSH-OUT SERVICES AND ELECTRONIC ALERT SERVICES

Although most of the search strategies and sites discussed previously require the user actively to enter their unique search query each time they are searching for information, so-called "push out services" and "electronic alert services" automatically update the user with new evidence as it is published. These services provide passive notification of new publications pertinent to the fields of interest selected by the user, at predetermined intervals or as soon as a relevant publication is indexed. Most of these services require entering a particular field of interest or keywords of interest, and a frequency at which updates are sent. For example, McMaster's MacPLUS service is a customized alerting service that updates clinicians without overwhelming their e-mail inboxes with low-precision search results. This service also includes clinicians in the ratings of relevance and newsworthiness. Although the service is currently designed for medicine, the rehabilitation version will be available in the next year (J. MacDermid, PT, PhD, personal communication, 2008). For hand surgeons, the subspecialties of orthopedic surgery and plastic surgery are listed as selection options.[19] Because the time and skill required to locate and appraise evidence is a major barrier to evidence-based practice, such "push-out" services provide a potential solution (**Table 3**).

LITERATURE SEARCH AT POINT OF CARE

Increasing numbers of clinicians are using handheld computers or personal digital assistants (PDAs) to access online medical evidence resources. The availability and portability of literature search and review and the integration of EBM

Table 3
Electronic alert services for evidence-based medicine

Web Site	URL	Description and Frequency
ACP Journal Club: Sentinel Reader Participatory Rating Service	http://www.acpjc.org/index.html	E-mailed links and reviews from American College of Physicians.
Amedeo	http://www.amedeo.com/	Allows choice of specialty interest areas, including "Surgery/Fractures," "Emergency Medicine," and "Rehabilitation Medicine." Biweekly.
BioMed Central	http://www.biomedcentral.com/	Open online publisher. Journals of interest include *BMC Surgery*, *Journal of Orthopedic Surgery*, and *Research and Pediatric Rheumatology*.
BMJ Updates McMaster University	http://bmjupdates.mcmaster.ca/ http://bmjupdates.mcmaster.ca/index.asp	*British Medical Journal* collaboration incorporating McMaster University's PLUS e-mail alerting system.
HighWire Press	http://highwire.stanford.edu/cgi/alerts	E-mail table of contents or new content with selected keywords. Offers RSS or personal digital assistant functionality for portable computers and web feeds. Includes *The Journal of Bone and Joint Surgery* and *Journal of Hand Surgery*.
MyNCBI	http://www.ncbi.nlm.nih.gov/entrez/query.fcgi?otool=nihlib	After registering and performing a PubMed search, click on "save search" link to receive e-mail updates of new search results.

resources at the point of care are some of the most enabling changes in modern medicine. PDAs are popular because of their ease-of-use, accessibility, and speed. Use of PDAs may be particularly helpful in researching medications at the point of care, including side effects and contraindications.[20] Some users prefer receiving updates of new resources by e-mail and some by alerts to their PDA (**Table 4**).[21]

PRACTICAL EXAMPLES AND SCENARIO

A 43-year-old patient comes to see you in the outpatient office. He has been diagnosed with lateral epicondylitis by his primary care physician. He has had the condition for the past 6 months. He works for the airline industry loading luggage. He denies any other medical illnesses. He has taken nonsteroidal drugs and has had one steroid injection. He searched the Internet and asks what the next step should be: rest, yoga, blood injections, physical therapy, transcutaneous electrical nerve stimulation, surgery, and so forth.

After completing a careful history and physical, the physician can proceed to do a literature search at the point of care. Using a PDA, the physician quickly elects to look up the BMJ Clinical Evidence Web site and review levels of evidence for each therapeutic modality. Alternatively, using a computer at point of care, the physician accesses the UpToDate Web site (http://www.uptodateonline.com) and enters "lateral epicondylitis" as the search term. A quick review of the "prognosis and refractory disease" section recommends further work-up with electrodiagnostic studies and consideration of surgical repair if pain persists after 1 year. Continued physical therapy with restriction of forearm use is also recommended.[22] The various options available are discussed with the patient using principles of shared decision-making. The patient agrees with a course of physical therapy and restriction of forearm use.

There is now time to perform a literature search on surgical treatments to keep updated on evidence-based support for surgical management.

Table 4
Evidence-based medicine resources for personal digital assistants

Resource	URL	Description
AvantGo	http://www.biomedcentral. com/info/about/avantgo	Research abstracts from BioMedCentral for personal digital assistants. Updated during personal digital assistant synchronization.
MD on TAP	http://mdot.nlm.nih.gov/proj/ mdot/mdot.php	Free utility from National Library of Medicine for searching Medline using a personal digital assistant.
PubMed for Handhelds Web Site	http://pubmedhh.nlm.nih.gov/ nlm/	Specially formatted Web site version of PubMed for display and use on personal digital assistants. Includes a population, intervention, comparison, outcome format search screen.

Using the PDA on the train ride home, the physician accesses the PubMed/MEDLINE Web site for PDAs by the population, intervention, comparison, and outcome methodology interface (http://pubmedhh.nlm.nih.gov/nlm/pico/piconew.html). The physician enters "chronic lateral epicondylitis" in the "medical condition" field, "male" as the "gender," "surgery" as the intervention, and "adult" in the "age group" field. Review of the results of the query produce one study evaluating the clinical and subjective functional results of open surgical treatment in patients with refractory lateral epicondylitis. The study is small (11 patients) and nonrandomized, underscoring the difficulty in finding RCTs for specialized clinical scenarios.[23] By the time the physician returns home, he or she is able to do a full literature review by PubMed, using the search term "lateral epicondylitis," clicking on "English" as the language, and "practice guideline" AND "review" as the types of study, published in the last year. The search produces a meta-review of RCTs of various surgical options for lateral epicondylitis and two reviews of current concepts in lateral epicondylitis.[24–26] Using institutional digital library access to the full-text versions of these articles, the physician is now ready to apply the critical tools in the rest of this volume to evaluation of the evidence.

THE FUTURE OF EVIDENCE RETRIEVAL

Once evidence is retrieved, it is time to review its quality and its applicability to the current clinical scenario. The quality of the search criteria theoretically can be calculated, using two systems-oriented evaluations. The first of these is recall, or the proportion of relevant documents retrieved from the database. The second of these is precision, or the proportion of relevant documents retrieved in the search.[27]

$$Recall = \frac{Retrieved\ documents\ that\ are\ relevant}{Relevant\ Documents}$$

$$Precision = \frac{Retrieved\ documents\ that\ are\ relevant}{Retrieved\ Documents}$$

Although recall and precision are theoretically important concepts for gauging the quality of search, they are often difficult if not impossible to calculate. This is because for a large database, such as MEDLINE, it is impossible to know the actual number of relevant documents (ie, "the golden standard" of search). It is likely that most clinical users are not concerned with how many relevant documents they miss or how many irrelevant ones they retrieve as long as they find the answer to their clinical question.[28] It is also reassuring that experienced clinicians are able to achieve comparable recall as professional librarians and better recall and precision than novice clinicians on their searches.[29]

The quality of evidence retrieved may be gauged through the use of one of several validated scales, including the Jadad and PEDro scales, the *Journal of Bone and Joint Surgery* scale, and Oxford Levels of Evidence. The scale developed by the *Journal of Bone and Joint Surgery* has been in use since 2003 and has been validated with low interrater variability.[30] Although numerous orthopedic journals currently report the Oxford Levels of Evidence, studies have shown variability in tier of quality between scales for the same research study.[31] Still, these validated scales of evidence provide the best estimation of study quality to the clinician interested in applying findings to a clinical scenario.

A metric known as the "journal's impact factor" has become a gauge of the journal's overall quality. An impact factor is a ratio between the numbers of citations in the current year of citable studies published in the journal in the past 2 years divided by the total number of citable studies published in the past 2 years.[32] The hand surgeon would likely be familiar with the journals that have the highest impact factors in the field. Caution must be exercised, however, in not assuming study quality simply because of the journal in which it appears. Impact factors are highly susceptible to falsely elevated values because of extreme specialization, self-citation, and citation density.[33] Familiarity with the commonly used criteria for study quality and careful reading of the study using statistical parameters, such as sensitivity, specificity, and number needed to treat, as is discussed elsewhere in this issue, are the best safeguards against integration of invalid evidence into practice. If this is impractical because of time constraints, then the publication's level-of-evidence score should be integral to the interpretation of the study's conclusion.

EBM is finding greater acceptance in surgical fields. International surveys of surgical practice have determined a steady move toward EBM. Among the features of orthopedic surgeons competent in EBM are younger age, experience of less than 10 years, possessing a PhD degree, and working in an academic setting. In one Dutch study, 27% of respondents used *Cochrane Reviews* in clinical decision-making.[34]

Another trend in EBM is integration of evidence resources at the point of care and into the medical record itself. Some electronic health record software packages and enterprise information systems now implement point of care InfoButtons or other formats of links to evidence-based resources relevant to the patient-specific information in the electronic health record.[35] Greater acceptance and use of such context-sensitive information retrieval methods is anticipated in the future, as better techniques for linking a specific patient scenario and search algorithms become available.

REFERENCES

1. Singer PA. Sex or survival: trade-offs between quality and quantity of life. J Clin Oncol 1991;9:328–34.

2. Kreder H. Evidence-based surgical practice: what is it and do we need it? World J Surg 1999;23:1232–5.

3. Giannoudis P, Bhandari M. Evidence-based medicine: what it is and what it is not. Injury 2006;37:302–6.

4. Surgical Outcomes Resource Centre. EBS surgery. Available at: http://www.fhs.mcmaster.ca/source/EBS/ebs-2.htm. Accessed March 23, 2008.

5. Amadio PC. What's new in hand surgery. J Bone Joint Surg Am 2008;89:453–8.

6. McKibbon A. PDQ evidence-based principles and practice. Hamilton (Canada): B.C. Decker; 1999.

7. Sackett DL. Evidence-based medicine: how to practice and teach EBM. Philadelphia: Churchill Livingstone; 2000.

8. Birch D, Eady A, Robertson D, et al. Users' guide to the surgical literature: how to perform a literature search. Can J Surg 2003;46:136–41.

9. National Library of Medicine. Stopwords. Available at: http://www.ncbi.nlm.nih.gov/books/bv.fcgi?highlight=stopwords&rid=helppubmed.table.pubmedhelp.T43. Accessed May 31, 2008.

10. Hersh W. Information retrieval, a health and biomedical perspective. New York: Springer-Verlag; 2003.

11. Wilczynski NL. Developing optimal search strategies for detecting clinically sound prognostic studies in MEDLINE: an analytic survey. BMC Med 2004;9:23.

12. American Academy of Orthopaedic Surgeons. American Academy of Orthopaedic Surgeons clinical guideline on diagnosis of carpal tunnel syndrome. Available at: http://www.aaos.org/Research/guidelines/CTS_guideline.pdf. Accessed March 24, 2008.

13. The Cochrane Collaboration. (2008, 5 31). Search Results. Available at: http://www.mrw.interscience.wiley.com/cochrane/cochrane_search_fs.html?mode=startsearch&products=all&unitstatus=all&opt1=OR&Query2=&zones2=article-title&opt2=AND&Query3=&zones3=author&opt3=AND&Query4=&zones4=abstract&opt4=AND&Query5=&zones5=tables&FromYea. Accessed May 31, 2008.

14. Brennan S, McKinin E. CINAHL and MEDLINE: a comparison of indexing practices. Bulletin of the American Library Association 1989;77:366–71.

15. Bhandari M, Montori VM, Devereaux PJ, et al. Doubling the impact: publication of systematic review articles in orthopaedic journals. J Bone Joint Surg Am 2004;86-A:1012–6.

16. Maher CG, Sherrington C, Herbert RD, et al. Reliability of the PEDro scale for rating quality of randomized controlled trials. Phys Ther 2003;83:713–21.

17. Bhogal S, Teasell R, Foley N, et al. The PEDro scale provides a more comprehensive measure of methodological quality than the Jadad Scale in stroke rehabilitation literature. J Clin Epidemiol 2005;58:668–73.

18. Johnson G, Cadwallader K, Scheffel S. Treatment of lateral epicondylitis. Am Fam Physician 2007;76:843–50.

19. McMaster University Heath Information Research Unit. Available at: http://hiru.mcmaster.ca/hiru/HIRU_McMaster_PLUS_Projects.aspx. Accessed August 3, 2008.

20. McCord G, Smucker WD, Selius BA, et al. Answering questions at the point of care: do residents practice EBM or manage information sources? Acad Med 2007;82:298–303.

21. Johnson ED, Pancoast PE, Mitchell JA, et al. Design and evaluation of a personal digital assistant-based alerting service for clinicians. J Med Libr Assoc 2004;92:438–44.

22. Anderson B, Sheon R. UpToDate. Epicondylitis. UpToDate. Available at: http://www.uptodateonline.com.novacat.nova.edu/online/content/topic.do?topicKey=ad_orth/6820&linkTitle=TREATMENT&source=preview&selectedTitle=1~11&anchor=14#14. Accessed February 5, 2008.

23. Işikan UE, Sarban S, Kocabey Y. The results of open surgical treatment in patients with chronic refractory lateral epicondylitis. Acta Orthop Traumatol Turc 2005;39:128–32.

24. Lo M, Safran M. Surgical treatment of lateral epicondylitis: a systematic review. Clin Orthop Relat Res 2007;Oct:98–106.

25. Calfee R, Patel A, DaSilva M, et al. Management of lateral epicondylitis: current concepts. J Am Acad Orthop Surg 2008;16:19–29.

26. Faro F, Wolf J. Lateral epicondylitis: review and current concepts. J Hand Surg [Am] 2007;463:98–106.

27. Hersh WS. Information retrieval and digital libraries. In: Shortliffe EC, editor. Biomedical informatics: computer applications in health care and biomedicine. New York: Springer; 2006. p. 660–97.

28. Harter S. Psychological relevance and information science. J Am Soc Inf Sci Technol 1992;43:602–15.

29. Haynes RM. Online access to MEDLINE in clinical settings. Ann Intern Med 1990;112:78–84.

30. Obremskey WT, Pappas N, Atallah-Wasif E, et al. Level of evidence in orthopaedic journals. J Bone Joint Surg Am 2005;87:2632–8.

31. Poolman RW, Struijs PAA, Krips R, et al. Does a level I evidence rating imply high quality of reporting in orthopaedic randomised controlled trials? BMC Med Res Methodol 2006;6:44.

32. Garfield E. Journal impact factors: a brief review. CMAJ 1999;161:979–80.

33. Hakkalamani S, Rawal A, Hennessy MS, et al. The impact factor of seven orthopaedic journals: factors influencing it. J Bone Joint Surg Br 2006;88:159–62.

34. Poolman R, Sierevelt I, Farrokhyar F, et al. Perceptions and competence in evidence-based medicine: are surgeons getting better? J Bone Joint Surg Am 2007;89:206–15.

35. Cimino JJ, Li J, Graham M, et al. Use of online resources while using a clinical information system. AMIA Annu Symp Proc 2003;175–9.

Critical Appraisal of Research Evidence for Its Validity and Usefulness

Joy C. MacDermid, BScPT, PhD[a,b,]*, David M. Walton, MScPT, PhD (c)[c],
Mary Law, PhD[d]

KEYWORDS

- Relevance • Clinical research • Critical appraisal
- Evidence-based • Quality • Clinical recommendations

FIVE STEPS OF EVIDENCE-BASED PRACTICE

The five steps in the evidence-based practice (EBP) approach are:

Ask a specific clinical question.
Find the best evidence to answer the question.
Critically appraise the evidence for its validity and usefulness.
Integrate appraisal results with clinical expertise and patient values.
Evaluate the outcomes.

Step 3 in the EBP approach involves critical appraisal of the validity and usefulness of evidence, with the specific goal of identifying the highest quality evidence that applies to a given clinical question. Because evidence-based decision making requires using the best available evidence, quality and relevance judgments are important components in the process. In fact, this third step can be broken down into three sequential subcomponents: (1) determine whether the results of individual studies are true (internally valid); (2) determine whether the results apply to a given patient (generalizability/external validity); and (3) determine the nature and strength of recommendations based on synthesis of several individual evidence resources.

Critical Appraisal of Individual Study Quality (Internal Validity)

The importance of critical appraisal in EBP has led to the development of systems, processes, tools, and support systems for rating clinical research evidence. In fact, we now have systematic reviews of appraisal tools.[1] In addition, there has been an increased move toward having experts in critical appraisal perform this task. Clinicians are then able to "pull-out" preappraised forms of evidence, such as the PEDro Physiotherapy Evidence Database or OTSeeker. Most recently, there has been development of "push-out" approaches, where high quality, critically appraised evidence resources already rated by experts are sent directly to end users with specific information needs (eg, BMJ updates). This article focuses on how hand surgeons and therapists can access and apply ranking systems, critical appraisal tools,

J.C.M. is funded by a New Investigator Award, Canadian Institutes of Health Research. D.M.W. is funded by a Doctoral Fellowship, Canadian Institutes of Health Research. M.L. holds the John and Margaret Lillie Chair in Childhood Disability.

[a] Hand and Upper Limb Centre Clinical Research Laboratory, St. Joseph's Health Centre, 268 Grosvenor Street, London, Ontario, N6A 4L6, Canada

[b] School of Rehabilitation Science, McMaster University, Institute for Applied Health Sciences, 1400 Main Street West, 4th Floor, Hamilton, Ontario L8S 1C7, Canada

[c] The University of Western Ontario School of Physical Therapy, Room EC 1588, 1201 Western Road, London, Ontario, N6G 1H1, Canada

[d] School of Rehabilitation Science, McMaster University, 268 Grosvenor Street, Hamilton, Ontario, Canada

* Corresponding author. School of Rehabilitation Science, LB33, McMaster University, Institute for Applied Health Sciences, Room 429, 1400 Main Street West, 4th Floor, Hamilton, Ontario L8S 1C7, Canada

E-mail address: macderj@mcmaster.ca (J.C. MacDermid).

Hand Clin 25 (2009) 29–42
doi:10.1016/j.hcl.2008.11.003

and guides for making overall recommendations to provide guideposts on how research evidence can be transitioned into patient specific recommendations.

Critical appraisal first focuses on the internal validity of the study, or the extent to which the conclusions of the study are true within the particular context of the study. This process can be performed at various depths of analysis, such as quick classification systems or more detailed rating tools. Critical appraisal instruments range from very structured tools that contain specific questions and defined response categories, to more open-ended scales where the assessor makes guided subjective judgments on the quality of aspects of study design, using a framework provided by the assessment tool. Different critical appraisal tools are appropriate for different study designs. Hand surgeons and therapists should select different critical appraisal instruments depending on their clinical question, its associated study design, their familiarity with critical appraisal, personal preferences, accessibility of the literature, and a realistic balance between time commitment and depth of analysis.

Different depths of critical appraisal are also appropriate at different points in practice. For example, when needing to make quick decisions at the point of care, screening for specific randomized, controlled trials (RCTs) or presynthesized evidence may be the most expedient approach. The classic five levels of evidence will be useful for this purpose. In other cases, when planning to implement a new intervention into one's practice, there may be a significant learning curve and cost involved. Therefore, it would be important to delve more deeply into the study design to gain a more thorough understanding of issues that might affect the validity of the study conclusions, and the clinical interpretability or applicability across different patients. Furthermore, knowing the evidence about a specific planned intervention can guide its implementation. Clinicians who commit to learning and practicing detailed critical appraisal gain a greater appreciation of the issues that can compromise confidence in research studies. However, quick rating scales or even presynthesized evidence ratings have the advantage of being less time consuming than more traditional evaluation methods.

LEVELS OF EVIDENCE

The concept of ranking levels of evidence is based on the principle that certain study types have more rigor and these higher quality study designs provide more confidence to associated clinical decision-making. The "best" study design varies according to the type of study that is being conducted. For example, while the RCT is considered the best study design for detecting differences between intervention groups, for studies in prognosis a prospective cohort design with complete follow-up is the best design. The types of study designs that have been used often signify the state of knowledge about an intervention. Early in the development of an intervention, case series are the most common. Data from these designs are then used to develop RCTs. The classic "Sacketts" five levels of evidence are a broad ordinal tool but have had a tremendous impact. For example, many evidence reviews performed by the Cochrane Collaboration include either only RCTs or the two highest levels of evidence when conducting a systematic review.

The "Classic" Levels of Evidence for Treatment Effectiveness

Because treatment effectiveness is one of the primary interests of clinicians, and the RCT is the ideal design for experimental evaluation of treatment effectiveness, the conduct of RCTs has expanded exponentially. Early evidence rating systems for treatment effectiveness designated RCTs as level 1 evidence. With the proliferation of RCTs emerged a new research methodology: the systematic review. The original levels of evidence developed at McMaster University were subsequently updated and are clearly presented on the Web site for the Oxford Center For Evidence-Based Medicine by David Sackett and colleagues (last updated May 2001, http://www.cebm.net/levels_of_evidence.asp). This rating system allows you to classify individual studies in broad categories or "levels" (see the article by Szabo and MacDermid elsewhere in this issue). Level 1 is the highest level of evidence that can be achieved for treatment effectiveness. Three potential situations are considered to be sufficiently rigorous to be labeled as level 1. Level 1a would consist of a systematic review of a number of RCTs, where the studies substantially agree with each other in terms of the direction and approximate size of the effects observed. A level 1b study would be an individual RCT where the size of the treatment effect was defined by a narrow confidence interval. A level 1c study is a very unusual circumstance in surgery or hand therapy, and is when an all-or-none phenomenon occurs in the absence of a randomized study. An example of a level 1c would be a study where an overwhelmingly dramatic change in outcomes can be demonstrated once a new treatment becomes available. Cases where all patients die before an intervention is available, and some survive following introduction up of a new intervention, provide overwhelming evidence. For example, vaccination is widely accepted in practice although not based on RCT evidence. Level 1 studies are those that provide the highest internal validity (confidence that the study results are true), enhancing our confidence that if we select this intervention for our patients, we will be able to achieve similar outcomes. These same levels pertain to studies of treatment effectiveness (therapy) prevention, etiology, and harm.

Fig. 1 illustrates how the levels of evidence hinge on a critical element important in research design. As we lose a critical element of internal validity, we also lose confidence that we might achieve the reported outcomes by selecting these interventions for our patients. Randomization is the single most protective factor against biases within clinical studies, as it controls for known and unknown confounders (assuming adequate sample size). Level 1 is the only level that provides experimental data, the remaining levels being observational.

Level 2 studies differ from RCTs in that we do not implement randomization. The protection against potential biases and confounders is lessened.[2] The most positive aspect of a prospective cohort study is that it identifies patients before experiencing the outcome (treatment or exposure), and thereby reduces the potential for a spectrum of biases (eg, differential recruitment, ascertainment bias, recall bias). A number of additional elements of research design are important to ensure that research designs maximize their

internal validity. These include the use of standardized outcome measures, adequate sampling, appropriate blinding,[3–5] rigorous follow-up, and proper statistical analysis, including adjustment for important potential confounders. A level 2a study is a systematic review of cohort (prospective) studies that agree with each other in terms of the direction and approximate size of the effects obtained. A level 2b study is a single, high quality cohort study (with greater than 80% follow-up). Follow-up is a critical element of quality, particularly in cohort studies where differential loss to follow-up might obliterate equality between groups, if it existed at the outset. Patients can drop out of studies because they experience overly favorable or unfavorable results compared with the remainder of the cohort. Thus, estimates of treatment effects may be over- or underestimated.

Level 3 studies for therapy are case-controlled designs. In a case-controlled study design, subgroups of patients are identified for study after their outcomes have been reached. Data collection about exposures, treatment options, and complications is retrospective. An example of such a design is a study of patients who did or did not return to work within 2 months following carpal tunnel surgery. Differences in these two groups of patients would be examined retrospectively to determine if treatment, or personal or work factors were associated with not returning to work. In case-controlled studies, we no longer have prospective data collection and are now subjected to additional sources of bias. For example, the authors experienced differential loss to follow-up in carpal tunnel surgery studies[6,7] where

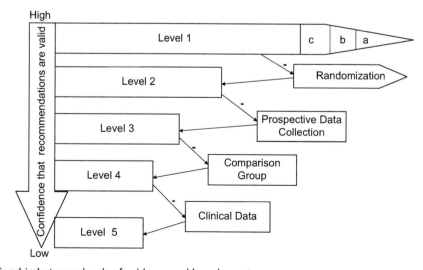

Fig. 1. Relationship between levels of evidence and key elements.

patients who were satisfied and had returned to work were reluctant to return for follow-up visits. Conversely, in another concurrent study on a different group of patients[8] (resection arthroplasty), the authors observed that patients who were dissatisfied were reluctant to return for a study visit determining final outcome status. The effect of dropouts on the estimated outcomes was different in these two cases. The reasons that specific subgroups of patients exist, are available for study, or provide specific outcomes data, are potentially related to the outcomes achieved (confounders) and can contaminate the observations.

At the next level of evidence another critical element of research design is lost: the comparison group. Level 4 evidence for treatment effectiveness consists of a single group or case series. No matter how rigorously we evaluate their outcomes, we remain uncertain what would have happened to these patients if an alternate intervention had been selected. Despite this flaw, case series remain one of the most common study designs reported in hand surgery journals,[9] and have, in some cases, been able to provide sufficient evidence to change practice, particularly where harm is demonstrated (eg, silicone synovitis). Investigators commonly attempt to mitigate the inherent weakness of this study design by comparing their results with those reported in other case series. However, these comparisons are tenuous because such a wide range of factors affect outcomes across settings.

Finally, at the lowest level of evidence, we lose the most critical component of internal validity when it comes to clinical research-observations made on patients. Level 5 consists of expert opinion, physiology, bench (laboratory) research, or first principles (eg, theory, anatomy, physiology, biomechanics). Although bench research, theory, and foundational science are very useful in generating hypotheses about what clinical outcomes might be achieved in specific clinical interventions, it is only through testing these hypotheses on actual patients that we have substantive evidence of the actual impact on patients.

Thus, one can see that the levels-of-evidence system is an ordinal ranking scale that focuses on the most critical element of research design for intervention studies.

Levels of Evidence for Other Study Designs

Other categories of clinical research require different study designs. Optimal designs for different clinical questions are specifically outlined in the table provided at the Center for Evidence-Based Medicine and included in the article "Introduction to evidence-based practice" by Szabo and MacDermid elsewhere in this issue. These include: prognosis, diagnosis, differential diagnosis/symptom prevalence study, economic, and decision analyses. For example, a level 1b for a prognosis study is an individual inception cohort study with greater than 80% follow-up, where a clinical decision rule has been validated in a single population. Conversely, the optimal study design for a diagnostic-test study consists of a cohort study with good reference standards or a clinical-decision rule tested within one clinical center. Despite differences in the optimal study design across different types of clinical questions, certain consistencies are evident:

A systematic review of high-quality studies always provides the highest level of rigor.
> An individual study using the optimal design for that type of clinical question is considered level 1.
> Prospective data collection indicates higher study quality than retrospective data collection.
> Expert opinion, bench research, conceptual frameworks/theories/first principles are always considered the lowest (level 5) evidence.

A variety of other rating systems have been proposed by different investigators. For example, different health service organizations have modified versions. Some of these organizations have used the term "levels of evidence" to refer to the overall state of evidence, whereas others use it for classifying individual studies. These systems may include different descriptors for five levels, the addition of different ranks (or subtypes), and even different labels.

While the intent of many of these investigators or organizations has been to simplify or customize processes to their needs, the existence of multiple systems provides an additional source of confusion. Despite this, there are many similarities across the different versions of the levels-of-evidence system. The authors prefer to use the classic five levels for ranking individual studies, as this is developed by leaders in the field, has been tested over many years, is relatively clear and comprehensive, is the most widely used system, and is easily accessible to the public (http://www.cebm.net/index.aspx?o=1025). The authors also choose to distinguish between the level of evidence of an individual study and the overall level of evidence that must be considered when making a recommendation. The latter involves synthesis of multiple studies and sources of evidence and is discussed in the "Grading recommendations" section later in this article.

Critical Appraisal Tools

While it is important to understand the basic principles involved in critical appraisal, the use of tools to provide structure to the process can be invaluable. All three authors have developed critical appraisal tools and use them for teaching critical appraisal or conducting systematic reviews or meta-analyses. Critical appraisal forms developed by Law and colleagues in 1998 are examples of open-ended critical appraisal tools. There are versions for intervention/effectiveness studies and qualitative studies. These tools can be downloaded from the McMaster University Web site at http://www.srs-mcmaster.ca/Default.aspx?tabid=630. The form and associated guide lead the appraiser to consider various aspects of design through a series of open-ended questions. These questions are listed in **Boxes 1, 2**.

A second type of critical appraisal approach is used by MacDermid. These tools provide structure with quantitative (3-point) response categories that are associated with specific descriptors for each item. Specific scoring criteria for each item are provided in an accompanying interpretation guide. Forms are available for effectiveness, diagnostic tests, and psychometric (outcome measure) studies. The forms and associated guides are available from the lead author (JM) and the questions included on each scale are listed in **Boxes 3–5**. One author (DW) developed a critical appraisal tool for prognostic studies to conduct a meta-analysis of studies on risk of poor outcomes following whiplash. The tool used items from the literature and other scales to derive the criteria judged most appropriate for this specific context (items in **Box 6**).

A variety of critical appraisal tools have been developed, and there is no clear indication which of them is best. There is debate amongst methodologists about the relative benefit of using customized critical appraisal tools or generic ones when conducting systematic reviews. For the purposes of improving your critical appraisal skills, it is important to discuss and compare your results with those derived by others. For example, the text *Evidence-Based Medicine: how to practice and teach EBM*, now comes with a CD containing a variety of examples from different types of articles and different disciplines.[10] The items used in the PEDro scale are sometimes used for critical appraisal in other

circumstances (http://www.pedro.fhs.usyd.edu.au/scale_item.html).

Many systematic reviews use the Jadad scale.[11] There are potential problems when using this scale to evaluate studies in hand surgery/therapy. First, two of the items relate to randomization, two relate to double blinding, and one relates to description of withdrawals and dropouts. Because hand surgery and hand therapy interventions do not easily lend themselves to double blinding, most studies fare poorly in quality ratings on this scale. For example, in a review of 2,169 published surgical trials in the *Journal of Bone and Joint Surgery* over a 10-year period, only 3% were randomized ($n = 64$). Of these, the overall mean study quality was 1.7/5.[12] Although a brief scale is preferable, there has been concern about the lack of comprehensive coverage of methodologic quality.[13] Second, there is a generalized concern about reliability of the scale,[12,14] especially among orthopedic surgeons.[12]

A systematic review addressed 120 different critical appraisal tools appearing in the literature.[1] This review found substantial variation between instruments in scope, structure, and scoring. **Table 1** provides additional Web sites that provide access to a variety of critical appraisal forms, and outline their purpose and number of items. Hand surgeons and therapists may wish to avoid scales designed only for use with RCTs (especially those that focus on blinding issues), as these will apply to only a small subset of the evidence currently available in the literature.

DO THE RESULTS APPLY TO MY PATIENT?

Once you decide that the conclusions within a given study are likely to be true, then you can move to the decision about relevance to your patient. You want to generalize results found within research studies for your patient. The basic question here is, "were the patients/circumstances in the study sufficiently similar to mine that my patient could reasonably expect a similar outcome?" You should know which aspects of your patient (disease, comorbidity, cultural, psychosocial, family, and so forth) will affect the outcomes of your test/intervention, and whether these were represented on the studied patients. Ideally, subgroup analyses within RCTs will highlight differential expectations for different subgroups.

You must also evaluate your own beliefs, skills, and circumstances to determine if they can reproduce the interventions studied in the literature. Critically evaluate your own expertise, equipment, staff, and setting: are there important differences,

Box 1
Critical review form—qualitative studies (Version 2.0)

Citation

Study purpose

1. Was the purpose and/or research question stated clearly? Outline the purpose of the study and/or research question.

Literature

2. Was relevant background literature reviewed?
3. Describe the justification of the need for this study. Was it clear and compelling?
4. How does the study apply to your practice and/or to your research question?
5. Is it worth continuing this review?

Study design

6. What was the design? Was the design appropriate for the study question? (ie, rationale) Explain.
7. Was a theoretic perspective identified? Describe the theoretic or philosophical perspective for this study: for example, researcher's perspective.
8. Describe the method(s) used to answer the research question. Are the methods congruent with the philosophical underpinnings and purpose?

Sampling

9. Was the process of purposeful selection described? Describe sampling methods used. Was the sampling method appropriate to the study purpose or research question?
10. Was sampling done until redundancy in data was reached? Are the participants described in adequate detail? How is the sample applicable to your practice or research question? Is it worth continuing?
11. Was informed consent obtained?

Data collection

12. Describe the context of the study. Was it sufficient for understanding of the "whole" picture?
13. What was missing and how does that influence your understanding of the research?
14. Do the researchers provide adequate information about data collection procedures (eg, gaining access to the site, field notes, training data gatherers)? Describe any flexibility in the design and data collection methods.

Data analyses

15. Describe method(s) of data analysis. Were the methods appropriate? What were the findings?
16. Describe the decisions of the researcher re: transformation of data to codes/themes. Outline the rationale given for development of themes.
17. Did a meaningful picture of the phenomenon under study emerge? How were concepts under study clarified and refined, and relationships made clear? Describe any conceptual frameworks that emerged.
18. Was there evidence of the four components of trustworthiness (credibility, transferability, dependability, confirmability)?
19. For each of the components of trustworthiness, identify what the researcher used to ensure each.
20. What meaning and relevance does this study have for your practice or research question?

Conclusions and implications

21. What did the study conclude? Were the conclusions appropriate given the study findings?
22. What were the main limitations of the study?
23. What were the implications of the findings for occupational therapy (practice and research)?

The full form and guide of this questionnaire (as well as an adapted word version) are available from: www.srs-mcmaster.ca/ResearchResour cesnbsp/CentreforEvidenceBasedRehabilitation/ EvidenceBasedPracticeResearchGroup/tabid/630/ Default.aspx

and if so, how might these modify your plan or expectations? Expert surgeons may achieve excellent outcomes with a complicated procedure they have performed hundreds of times, but novice surgeons are unlikely to get similar outcomes. This is particularly true for more complex surgical skills, such as arthroscopic techniques. Similarly, some specialized rehabilitation therapies are highly effective with advanced training but similar outcomes may not be achieved without the same level of training and experience. This is particularly true for more complex technical skills, such as manual therapies or complicated orthotic devices.

Box 2
Critical review form—quantitative studies

Citation

Study purpose

1. Was the purpose and/or research question stated clearly? Outline the purpose of the study and/or research question.

Literature

2. Was relevant background literature reviewed?
3. Describe the justification of the need for this study.

Design

4. Describe the study design. Was the design appropriate for the study question? (eg, for knowledge level about this issue, outcomes, ethical issues, and so forth).
5. Specify any biases that may have been operating and the direction of their influence on the results.

Sample

6. Was the sample described in detail (who, characteristics, how many, how was sampling done?) If more than one group, was there similarity between the groups?
7. Was the sample size justified?
8. Describe ethics procedures. Was informed consent obtained?

Outcomes

9. Were the outcome measures reliable?
10. Were the outcome measures valid?
11. Specify the frequency of outcome measurement (ie, pre-, post-, follow-up), the outcome areas and list the measures that were used.

Intervention

12. Was the intervention described in detail?
13 Provide a short description of the intervention (focus, who delivered it, how often, setting). Could the intervention be replicated in practice?
14. Was contamination avoided?
15. Was cointervention avoided?

Results

16. Were results reported in terms of statistical significance?
17. What were the results? Were they statistically significant (ie, $P<.05$)? If not statistically significant, was study big enough to show an important difference if it should

occur? If there were multiple outcomes, was that taken into account for the statistical analysis?
18. Were the analysis methods appropriate?
19. What was the clinical importance of the results? Were differences between groups clinically meaningful? (if applicable)
20. Did any participants drop out from the study? Why? (Were reasons given and were drop-outs handled appropriately?)

Conclusions and implications

21. What did the study conclude?
22. What are the implications of these results for practice? What were the main limitations or biases in the study?
23. Were the conclusions appropriate given the study methods and results?

The full form and guide of this questionnaire (as well as an adapted word version) are available from: www.srs-mcmaster.ca/ResearchResour cesnbsp/CentreforEvidenceBasedRehabilitation/ EvidenceBasedPracticeResearchGroup/tabid/630/ Default.aspx

Courtesy of the Evidence-Based Practice Research Group, McMaster University, Hamilton, ON; with permission. Copyright © 1998.

Grading Recommendations

While the levels-of-evidence system provides the user with a relative level of confidence in the results of individual study findings, making practice recommendations based on all available evidence in an area is often challenging for the novice evidence-based practitioner, as less attention has been directed at this process. The process involves examining multiple studies to make overall recommendations. Grades of A to D, which focused primarily on the level of evidence, have been commonly used (http:// www.cebm.net/index.aspx?o=1025). One disadvantage of this system is that it focuses primarily on the nature of the evidence and does not consider other factors that would influence the strength of recommendations. Perhaps for this reason, a variety of systems and scales have been developed for grading recommendations. A further complication is that these recommendation scales have varied widely across different organizations, as organizations try to develop systems that meet their individual needs. For example, some have altered the terminology, some prefer visual indicators, and some include different conceptual components (eg, balance of risk and harm or costs) in the recommendation process.

Box 3
Critical appraisal of study design for psychometric articles evaluation items (outcome measure research)

Evaluation criteria

Study question

1. Was the relevant background research cited to define what is currently known about the psychometric properties of the measures under study, and the need or potential contributions of the current research question?

Study design

2. Were appropriate inclusion/exclusion criteria defined?
3. Were specific psychometric hypotheses identified?
4. Was an appropriate scope of psychometric properties considered?
5. Was an appropriate sample size used?
6. Was appropriate retention/follow-up obtained? (Studies involving retesting or follow-up only)

Measurements

7. Documentation: Were specific descriptions provided or referenced that explain the measures and its correct application/interpretation (to a standard that would allow replication)?
8. Standardized methods: Were administration and application of measurement techniques within the study standardized and did they consider potential sources of error/misinterpretation?

Analyses

9. Were analyses conducted for each specific hypothesis or purpose?
10. Were appropriate statistical tests conducted to obtain point estimates of the psychometric property?
11. Were appropriate ancillary analyses were done to describe properties beyond the point estimates (Confidence intervals, benchmark comparisons, standard error of measurement/minimal important difference)?

Recommendations

12. Were the conclusions/clinical recommendations supported by the study objectives, analysis and results?

Total score % (sum of subtotals/24*100) is based on criteria met from the rating guide and scored as 2,1, or 0 depending on compliance with standards.

This Box lists the criteria rating the quality of a study addressing the psychometric properties of an outcome measure. The full form and guide are available from the author or in the textbook *Evidence-Based Rehabilitation*.

Courtesy of Joy C. MacDermid, BScPT, PhD, London, ON. Copyright © 2008; used with permission.

For example, an overall rating of evidence across different studies is used by some medical groups and contains just four levels (obtained from http://www.cochranemsk.org/review/writing): platinum, gold, silver, and bronze. This system gives qualitative ratings based on number and quality (based on two or three key criteria), as listed below. Note that two of the four levels require RCTs. Within this system, case series are demoted to the lowest level of evidence, with expert opinion and bench research, and there is less differential between cohort/case-controlled designs. For hand surgery, this system is likely to rank most current evidence at the lowest level. The authors do not recommend this option for surgery, primarily because the authors believe a better approach is evolving to consensus (see the Grades Of Recommendation Assessment, Development and Evaluation Working Group or GRADE).

Platinum level
The platinum ranking is given to evidence that meets the following criteria as reported in a published systematic review that has at least two individual controlled trials, each satisfying the following:

Sample sizes of at least 50 per group. If they do not find a statistically significant difference, they are adequately powered for a 20% relative difference in the relevant outcome.
Blinding of patients and assessors for outcomes;
Handling of withdrawals greater than 80% follow-up—imputations based on methods such as last observation carried forward acceptable;
Concealment of treatment allocation.

Gold level
The gold ranking is given to evidence if at least one RCT meets all of the following criteria as reported:

Sample sizes of at least 50 per group. If they do not find a statistically significant difference, they are adequately powered for

Box 4
Criteria for evaluation of quality of an intervention study

Evaluation criteria

Study question

1. Was the relevant background work cited to establish a foundation for the research question?

Study design

2. Was a comparison group used?
3. Was patient status at more than 1 time point considered?
4. Was data collection performed prospectively?
5. Were patients randomized to groups?
6. Were patients blinded to the extent possible?
7. Were treatment providers blinded to the extent possible?
8. Was an independent evaluator used to administer outcome measures?

Subjects

9. Did sampling procedures minimize sample/selection biases?
10. Were inclusion/exclusion criteria defined?
11. Was an appropriate enrollment obtained?
12. Was appropriate retention/follow-up obtained?

Intervention

13. Was the intervention applied according to established principles?
14. Were biases due to the treatment provider minimized (ie, attention, training)?
15. Was the intervention compared with an appropriate comparator?

Outcomes

16. Was an appropriate primary outcome defined?
17. Were appropriate secondary outcomes considered?
18. Was an appropriate follow-up period incorporated?

Analysis

19. Was an appropriate statistical test(s) performed to indicate differences related to the intervention?
20. Was it established that the study had significant power to identify treatment effects?

21. Was the size and significance of the effects reported?
22. Were missing data accounted for and considered in analyses?
23. Were clinical and practical significance considered in interpreting results?

Recommendations

24. Were the conclusions/clinical recommendations supported by the study objectives, analysis and results?

Total Quality Score based on sum of above (2,1, or 0 per item) =/48.
Level of Evidence (Sackett) 1 ☐ 2 ☐ 3☐ 4☐ 5☐. This figure lists the criteria rating the quality of a study addressing effectiveness. It can be used for all levels of studies. The reviewer is also given a checkbox to mark the level according to the classic levels of evidence rating system. The items are scored 2,1,0. The full form and guide are available from the author or in textbook *Evidence-Based Rehabilitation*.

Courtesy of Joy C. MacDermid, BScPT, PhD, London, ON. Copyright © 2008; used with permission.

a 20% relative difference in the relevant outcome.

Blinding of patients and assessors for outcomes;

Handling of withdrawals greater than 80% follow-up—imputations based on methods such as last observation carried forward acceptable;

Concealment of treatment allocation.

Silver level

The silver ranking is given to evidence if a systematic review or randomized trial does not meet the above criteria. Silver ranking would also include evidence from at least one study of nonrandomised cohorts who did and did not receive the therapy or evidence from at least one case-controlled study. A randomized trial with a "head-to-head" comparison of agents is considered silver level ranking unless a reference is provided to a comparison of one of the agents to placebo showing at least a 20% relative difference.

Bronze level

The bronze ranking is given to evidence if there is at least one high-quality case series without controls (including simple before and after studies in which the patient acts as their own control) or if it is derived from expert opinion based on clinical experience without reference to any of the foregoing (for example, argument from physiology, bench research or first principles).

In fact, there is little consistency across these rating systems and limitations have been noted.[15] This lack of consistency can make it difficult for the inexperienced evidence-based practitioner to understand how they should deal with multiple pieces of information. This is particularly problematic when groups try to develop evidence-based clinical practice guidelines where the strength and wording of the recommendations are a key output. In response to this concern, an international group, the GRADE Working Group, focused on development of a system that could be used to grade the quality of evidence and strength of

Table 1
Online critical appraisal/recommendations tools

Web Site URL	Type of Studies Evaluated	Number of Items
Appraisal of Guidelines for Research & Evaluation[a] http://www.agreecollaboration.org/	Clinical practice guidelines	23
Best Evidence Topics http://www.bestbets.org/links/BET-CA-worksheets.php	Diagnostic test Economic analysis Prognosis Systematic review Qualitative research Clinical practice guidelines	29 34 37 33 40 32
Center for Evidence Based Emergency Medicine http://www.ebem.org/analyse.html	Treatment effectiveness Prognosis Diagnostic test Systematic review	13 10 11 12–15
Center for Evidence Based Medicine, Oxford http://www.cebm.net/critical_appraisal.asp	Treatment effectiveness Prognosis Diagnostic test Economic analysis Systematic review Clinical practice guidelines	11 10 8 14 10 18
Center for Health Evidence[a] http://www.cche.net/usersguides/main.asp	Treatment effectiveness Diagnostic test Prognosis Clinical practice guideline Economic analysis Qualitative research	12 9 9 10 10 8
Critical Appraisal Skills Program[a] http://www.phru.nhs.uk/Pages/PHD/resources.htm	Diagnostic test Qualitative study Economic analysis Systematic review	12 10 10 10
Evidence Based Medicine, Alberta[a] http://www.med.ualberta.ca/ebm/ebm.htm	Treatment effectiveness Prognosis Diagnostic test Economic analysis Systematic review Clinical practice guidelines	11 10 10 10 11 11
Evidence Based Medicine, Duke http://www.mclibrary.duke.edu/subject/ebm?tab=appraising&extra=worksheets	Treatment effectiveness Prognosis Diagnostic test Qualitative study Economic analysis Systematic review Clinical practice guidelines	12 9 9 7 10 10 4
Health Care Practice Research & Development Unit http://www.fhsc.salford.ac.uk/hcprdu/critical-appraisal.htm	Treatment effectiveness Qualitative study Economic analysis	51 44 68
McMaster—School of Rehabilitation Science[a] http://www.srs-mcmaster.ca/ResearchResourcesnbsp/CentreforEvidenceBasedRehabilitation/EvidenceBasedPracticeResearchGroup/tabid/630/Default.aspx	Treatment effectiveness Qualitative study	15 27

(continued on next page)

Table 1
(continued)

Web Site URL	Type of Studies Evaluated	Number of Items
Quality of Reporting of Meta-analyses http://www.consort-statement.org/ QUOROM.pdf	Systematic review	17
School of Health and Related Research (ScHARR), University of Sheffield[a] http://www.shef.ac.uk/scharr/sections/ir/ links	Systematic review Qualitative study	10 10
GRADE Working Group http://www. gradeworkinggroup.org/	Documents and free software supporting use of GRADE approach to making recommendations	—

[a] Has guide to interpretation.

recommendations in a method that balanced simplicity and clarity.[15–23] A number of articles have subsequently been published on their consensus of how to rate quality of evidence and strength of recommendations.

The GRADE system classifies evidence in one of four levels: high, moderate, low, or very low. Evidence is considered high quality if further research is very unlikely to change our confidence in the estimate of the effects. Moderate quality is present if further research is likely to have an important impact on our confidence in the estimate of the effect and may actually change the estimate. If further research is very likely to have an important impact on our confidence in the estimate of the effect and is likely to change the estimate, then it is considered low quality. If the estimated effect is very uncertain, the quality of evidence is considered very low quality.

Evidence based on RCTs starts off as high quality evidence but can decrease to a lower level if there are significant study limitations, inconsistency of results, indirectness of the evidence, imprecision, or reporting bias. Observational studies start off as low quality that can be graded upwards if the magnitude of the treatment effect is very large, or if all plausible sources of confounding have been identified and controlled, or if there is evidence of a dose-response gradient. Because various groups have in the past conveyed quality of evidence in different formats, there are nonspecific recommendations for using letters, numbers, symbols, and words to communicate grades of evidence. For example, high quality evidence can be labeled using the word "high," or alternatively, the number "1," the letter "A," the full darkened circle symbol "●" or the star approach "★ ★ ★ ★."[24] There

have been suggestions that clinicians respond more favorably to symbols than they do to numbers or letters.[25]

There are four factors that influence the strength of the recommendation. Of these, the quality of evidence is one factor. The higher the quality of evidence, the more likely a strong recommendation is warranted. Strong recommendations tend to use statements that are in that category of "definitely should do" or "definitely should not do." Secondly, the balance between desirable and undesirable effects is considered. The larger the difference between desirable and undesirable effects, the more likely a strong recommendation is warranted. The narrower this gradient, the more likely a weak recommendation is warranted. For example, in hand surgery there has been considerable controversy about the relative role of endoscopic versus open carpal tunnel release. Despite numerous RCTs and systematic reviews and meta-analyses, there remains controversy. Part of this controversy is related to the fact that even in well-designed studies, the differential effects are narrow. Therefore, regardless of the quality of evidence, only weak recommendations should be made on use of these two interventions.

Weak recommendations tend to be more in the category of "probably should (or should not) do," and allow more latitude for the individual practitioner to consider local circumstances as potentially outweighing the small differential in potential effectiveness. For example, a more appropriate recommendation for carpal tunnel surgery might be that surgeons should examine a summary of evidence comparing endoscopic and open carpal tunnel release and be aware that there is strong evidence of small differential outcomes between the two procedures. Differential outcomes include the potential for faster return to work and slightly higher (but still low) risk of complications with endoscopic procedures, as well as small differential recovery in physical impairments. Surgeons should be prepared to consider and discuss with patients their own experience, expertise, and circumstances, and the patient's values and preferences to choose the best surgical option.

A third factor that influences the strength of recommendation concerns patient values and preferences. The more variable or uncertain values and preferences are, the more likely a weak recommendation should be used. Finally, costs and resource allocation can be considered. The higher the cost of an intervention (particularly when considering cost:benefit ratio) the less likely a strong recommendation is warranted.

The GRADE system offers two grades of recommendation—strong and weak—and an option for no specific recommendation when the trade-offs are equally balanced or uncertain. When the desirable effects of intervention clearly outweigh the undesirable effects (or clearly do not), then strong recommendations are warranted. When trade-offs are less certain, the quality of evidence is lower, values are uncertain, or resource use is a concern, then the relative desirability may be less certain. Thus, the grades are 1 (strong), 2 (weak), or 0 (no specific recommendation).

Practitioners may find it helpful to record their evidence-based conclusions in short one-page summaries. The Center for Evidence-Based Medicine provides a free downloadable "CAT-maker" that calculates the number needed-to-treat from study data and allows one to summarize the available evidence on a one-page summary in a standardized fashion that can be stored in a personal file of evidence reviews (http://www.cebm.net/index.aspx?o=1216). Once the hand surgeon or therapist is clear in his or her own mind about the overall balance of the research evidence and has formulated that into a recommendation that they are comfortable with, they can then move to the process of integrating their view with the patients. The process of incorporating patient-centered care or shared decision-making with the evidence and clinical experience has been highlighted in other articles in this issue. A critical analysis of the literature and formulation of clear recommendations makes it easier to communicate more effectively with patients during these discussions. See Appendix 1 for useful Web links regarding the ideas discussed in this article.

APPENDIX 1: USEFUL WEB LINKS

http://bmjupdates.mcmaster.ca/index.asp (BMJ updates): A free push service (through McMaster University and BMJ) that delivers customized appraised research by email in the content areas and frequency you request.

http://davidmlane.com/hyperstat/index.html: Free online statistics textbook.

http://nilesonline.com/stats: Easy reading statistics textbook.

http://statpages.org: Free online statistics calculations.

http://www.cebm.net/critical_appraisal.asp (Center for Evidence-Based Medicine, Oxford): This site provides a database of critically appraised topics and tools.

http://www.consort-statement.org (Homepage): The CONSORT statement lays out a number of guidelines for conducting good RCTs, which are essential for sound systematic reviews. The homepage has more detailed information and updates on current work.

http://www.otseeker.com (OTseeker): This is a searchable database that provides abstracts and ratings of RCTs and systematic reviews relevant to occupational therapy.

http://www.pedro.fhs.usyd.edu.au (PEDro): This is a searchable Physiotherapy Evidence Database that provides bibliographic details, abstracts, and ratings of RCTs, systematic reviews, and evidence-based clinical practice guidelines in physiotherapy.

http://www.sportsci.org/resource/stats/index.html: An excellent primer or refresher to many aspects of statistics, complied and created by New Zealander William Hopkins.

REFERENCES

1. Katrak P, Bialocerkowski AE, Massy-Westropp N, et al. A systematic review of the content of critical appraisal tools. BMC Med Res Methodol 2004;4: 22.

2. Mamdani M, Sykora K, Li P, et al. Reader's guide to critical appraisal of cohort studies: 2. Assessing potential for confounding. BMJ 2005;330(7497): 960–2.

3. Montori VM, Bhandari M, Devereaux PJ, et al. In the dark: the reporting of blinding status in randomized controlled trials. J Clin Epidemiol 2002;55(8): 787–90.

4. Devereaux PJ, Bhandari M, Montori VM, et al. Double blind, you are the weakest link–goodbye!. Equine Vet J 2005;37(6):557–8.

5. Devereaux PJ, Bhandari M, Montori VM, et al. Double blind, you have been voted off the island! Evid Based Ment Health 2002;5(2):36–7.

6. MacDermid JC, Richards RS, Roth JH, et al. Endoscopic versus open carpal tunnel release: a randomized trial. J Hand Surg [Am] 2003;28(3):475–80.

7. Boyd KU, Gan BS, Ross DC, et al. Outcomes in carpal tunnel syndrome: symptom severity, conservative management and progression to surgery. Clin Invest Med 2005;28(5):254–60.

8. Bain GI, Pugh DM, MacDermid JC, et al. Matched hemiresection interposition arthroplasty of the distal radioulnar joint. J Hand Surg [Am] 1995;20(6):944–50.

9. Amadio PC, Higgs P, Keith M. Prospective comparative clinical trials in the journal of hand surgery (American). J Hand Surg [Am] 1996;21(5):925–9.

10. Sackett DL, Straus SE, Richardson WS, et al. Evidence-based medicine. How to practice and teach EBM. 2nd edition. Toronto: Churchill Livingstone; 2000.

11. Jadad AR, Moore RA, Carroll D, et al. Assessing the quality of reports of randomized clinical trials: is blinding necessary? Control Clin Trials 1996;17(1):1–12.

12. Bhandari M, Richards RR, Sprague S, et al. Quality in the reporting of randomized trials in surgery: is the Jadad scale reliable? Control Clin Trials 2001; 22(6):687–8.

13. Bhogal SK, Teasell RW, Foley NC, et al. The PEDro scale provides a more comprehensive measure of methodological quality than the Jadad scale in stroke rehabilitation literature. J Clin Epidemiol 2005;58(7):668–73.

14. Clark HD, Wells GA, Huet C, et al. Assessing the quality of randomized trials: reliability of the Jadad scale. Control Clin Trials 1999;20(5):448–52.

15. Atkins D, Eccles M, Flottorp S, et al. Systems for grading the quality of evidence and the strength of recommendations I: critical appraisal of existing approaches The GRADE Working Group. BMC Health Serv Res 2004;4(1):38.

16. Atkins D, Best D, Briss PA, et al. Grading quality of evidence and strength of recommendations. BMJ 2004;328(7454):1490.

17. Atkins D, Briss PA, Eccles M, et al. Systems for grading the quality of evidence and the strength of recommendations II: pilot study of a new system. BMC Health Serv Res 2005;5(1):25.

18. Guyatt G, Baumann M, Pauker S, et al. Addressing resource allocation issues in recommendations from clinical practice guideline panels: suggestions from an American College of Chest Physicians task force. Chest 2006;129(1):182–7.

19. Guyatt G, Vist G, Falck-Ytter Y, et al. An emerging consensus on grading recommendations? ACP J Club 2006;144(1):A8–9.

20. Guyatt G, Gutterman D, Baumann MH, et al. Grading strength of recommendations and quality of evidence in clinical guidelines: report from an American College of Chest Physicians task force. Chest 2006;129(1):174–81.

21. Guyatt GH, Oxman AD, Kunz R, et al. Going from evidence to recommendations. BMJ 2008; 336(7652):1049–51.

22. Guyatt GH, Oxman AD, Vist GE, et al. GRADE: an emerging consensus on rating quality of evidence and strength of recommendations. BMJ 2008; 336(7650):924–6.

23. Guyatt GH, Oxman AD, Kunz R, et al. Incorporating considerations of resources use into grading recommendations. BMJ 2008;336(7654):1170–3.

24. Schunemann HJ, Best D, Vist G, et al. Letters, numbers, symbols and words: how to communicate grades of evidence and recommendations. CMAJ 2003;169(7):677–80.

25. Akl EA, Maroun N, Guyatt G, et al. Symbols were superior to numbers for presenting strength of recommendations to health care consumers: a randomized trial. J Clin Epidemiol 2007;60(12): 1298–305.

Diagnosis, Diagnostic Criteria, and Consensus

Brent Graham, MD, MSc, FRCSC*

KEYWORDS

- Diagnosis • Diagnostic criteria • Consensus
- Measurement scales • Clinical disagreement

The focus in much of the medical literature is on the outcome of treatment. It is implicitly assumed that the diagnoses leading to the treatments under scrutiny are always accurate. However, most seasoned clinicians recognize that where treatment is unsuccessful an inaccurate diagnosis may be as likely the cause of the treatment failure as ineffectiveness of the intervention itself. Despite this, there has been comparatively little attention paid to the process of diagnosis[1] beyond the description of new technologies, such as those in imaging. This is a potentially serious problem because it is very clear that diagnostic inaccuracy is an inevitable occurrence and it is possible that it is substantially more common and costly than most clinicians suspect.[2]

DIAGNOSTIC TESTS AND DIAGNOSTIC SCALES

If the process of diagnosis is thought of as a form of measurement then it is possible that it can be made more consistent by using diagnostic scales, just as outcome measurement scales can standardize the results of treatment. The development of diagnostic scales can follow the usual approaches of measurement theory and should have the same advantages of outcome instruments that are created using these concepts, namely reliability and validity. The importance of this cannot be overstated. If the criteria used to make a diagnosis are unreliable or are inconsistently applied then the selection of treatment becomes as dependent on where the diagnosis is made or who makes it as it is on the diagnostic label itself. For the individual patient this is obviously problematic because it follows that treatment will vary with the setting in which it takes place and

this contradicts the whole concept of evidence-based care; namely that the identification of the best treatments should be based on knowledge and knowledge alone. There are also ramifications for the health care system at large if diagnostic inaccuracies are widespread because the prevalence of various diseases, identified in the databases of large health care systems as diagnoses, would be expected to at least partially inform policy making by both government and insurers.[3]

A familiar example for hand surgeons would be that of carpal tunnel syndrome (CTS). This condition is diagnosed by a wide range of clinicians including orthopaedic surgeons, plastic surgeons, neurosurgeons, neurologists, rheumatologists, physiatrists, and a variety of primary care physicians including family doctors and occupational health physicians. While it may be assumed that the same diagnostic criteria are used for this common clinical entity by doctors working in these widely divergent specialties, in fact agreement on the best clinical criteria for the diagnosis is low both within and across these groups.[4] An inaccurate diagnosis of CTS may lead to inappropriate treatment or, conversely, inadequate treatment if the diagnosis is not made when the condition is present. Inconsistency in diagnostic practices may also suggest an association with certain exposures, such as those in a given workplace, which may be completely spurious.

Improving the reliability of diagnoses can be achieved in a number of ways starting with increasing the number of criteria used to make a particular diagnosis. This is a familiar concept in educational testing. It is clear that the more items there are on a test the more reliable the test in reflecting the attainment of the individual. Simply

University of Toronto, University Health Network Hand Program, Toronto, Ontario, Canada
* Toronto Western Hospital, 399 Bathurst Street, 2E-425, Toronto, Ontario M5T 2S8, Canada.
E-mail address: brent.graham@uhn.on.ca

Hand Clin 25 (2009) 43–48
doi:10.1016/j.hcl.2008.10.004
0749-0712/08/$ – see front matter © 2009 Published by Elsevier Inc.

stated, if it looks like a duck, sounds like a duck, and feels like a duck, it is more reliably a duck than if it only looks like a duck.

The use of a large number of items characterizes most outcome instruments, which usually measure a number of constructs that have an impact on the result. A scale that simply asked "Are you better than before treatment?" would not be very useful because this is too much of a summation and does not take into account discomfort, morbidity, cost, and other factors that might be important in defining treatment as successful. As a result, this approach, though attractive in its simplicity, does not necessarily answer the question of whether treatment has been effective. Similarly, in the process of making a diagnosis it is assumed that elements of the clinical evaluation including the history and physical examination, and laboratory tests will be used in establishing the diagnosis. Just as in the development of outcome measures, determining what a diagnostic scale should include should involve a process of item generation, item reduction and then testing for reliability and validity.

Clearly this type of approach is not always required. The diagnosis of a fractured femur can be easily deduced simply by looking at the injured limb and obtaining a radiograph. However, where an element of judgment is required to make a correct diagnosis there may be a need for the integration of more and varied information. The process of considering different findings, assigning a certain amount of importance to each finding, and summarizing the accumulated meaning of the available information certainly occurs implicitly as most experienced clinicians make their analysis. However, translating that intuitive process into an operational instrument like a diagnostic scale may increase the ability of nonexpert clinicians to make the same diagnoses, prevent experienced diagnosticians from making mistakes, and lead to greater consistency in the establishment of diagnoses.

To take up the example of CTS again, in many instances the diagnosis will be made primarily or even exclusively on the basis of the result of electrodiagnostic testing. Where these tests are interpreted as positive, the clinical evaluation may be completely trumped by the test result if the importance of electrodiagnostic testing is heavily weighted in the diagnostic process. Conversely, definitive treatment, like surgical decompression, may be delayed or withheld altogether if the electrodiagnostic tests are considered negative, even where there are substantial clinical findings to suggest the diagnosis. Clearly a combination of findings from the history, physical examination, and electrodiagnostic data, interpreted in the context of the clinical evaluation, provides the most information on which to make a diagnostic conclusion. The way in which this data is weighted and integrated could be seen as a reflection of clinical expertise; however, there have been attempts to model the evaluation to improve the consistency of diagnoses made by nonexperts in the field.[5]

Here it may be useful to briefly examine the difference between a diagnostic test and a diagnostic scale. For some conditions, a diagnostic test, usually based on a laboratory finding (for the purposes of this discussion these will be considered synonymous), will be the basis of a diagnosis. A simple example would be the diagnosis of streptococcal pharyngitis based on a positive culture from a throat swab. However, there are many conditions where data obtained from testing does not so much identify the diagnosis as give insight into severity, response to treatment, and prognosis.[6] For these conditions, the collection of laboratory data might be seen as complementing clinically acquired data from the history and physical examination. Where the relative importance of clinical and laboratory data can be quantified, it may be possible to develop an instrument that can be used to identify the condition; in other words, a diagnostic scale. The inherent attraction of such an instrument is in the potential for consistently using the most pertinent and useful criteria regardless of who is making the evaluation. Implicit in this idea is the assumption that the history or physical examination maneuvers can be performed with the same reliability by experts and nonexperts alike. This is not necessarily true, nor should it be expected that there is no role for the kind of clinical judgment that characterizes expertise. But the opportunity to standardize diagnostic criteria wherever this is feasible should be expected to lead to improvements and efficiencies in the selection and implementation of treatments.

HOW SHOULD A DIAGNOSTIC SCALE BE CREATED?

The development of any measurement scale should follow three basic steps: item generation, item reduction, and psychometric testing (ie, evaluation of the reliability and validity of the instrument). In addition to these basic steps, the determination of the actual usefulness of any scale requires a consideration of characteristics such as responsiveness and sensibility, which are beyond the scope of the present discussion.[7]

The goal of item generation is to identify any and all factors that might be pertinent to the subject of the scale. In the case of a diagnostic scale, this might include items from the clinical history and physical examination as well as laboratory data. It is very important that this search be comprehensive so that any potentially important items are not excluded from consideration. The published literature and textbooks are an important starting point for this process because these sources represent what is commonly known about the topic. Beyond this, however, it may be important to consult experts in the clinical area. These individuals often have insights into the subject that are based on their experience and which do not necessarily find their way into the mainstream medical literature.

Once the pool of potential items for inclusion in the scale has been identified, the next step is to decide which should be included and which should be discarded. A balance has to be maintained between comprehensiveness and feasibility. Clearly the larger the number of items used to make the measurement, the more reliable the information provided by the scale, whether related to the characterization of an outcome or a diagnosis. However, if there are too many items then the instrument will be unwieldy and will be unlikely to achieve acceptance. The actual number of items that is ideal for a given scale depends in large measure on the goal and this is a decision for the developers of the instrument to consider. The actual process of reducing the item pool to the appropriate number may require a number of approaches. These might include judgments of a panel of experts[8] or any of a number of statistical approaches such as principle components analysis. Again, the details around this topic are beyond the scope of this article, but there is an abundant amount of information about the various approaches contained within the methodologic literature.[7]

Once item reduction has been completed, the prototype scale will be established. In some instances, some of the items will be given more weight than others. This may be established during the item reduction phase if a statistical approach is used. In other cases, the diagnostic items may have the equal importance. This will often depend on the condition being studied or on the objective of creating the scale. The next step is to determine if the scale is reliable and valid. The methods for establishing reliability are varied, but the principle that has to be understood is that it is critical that the scale perform in a consistent manner regardless of the setting in which it is used or the identity of observer implementing the instrument. These goals have to be considered in planning testing of the instrument for reliability. For example, if the objective is to standardize the diagnosis of a common condition like CTS, then it makes sense to test the instrument in a setting where CTS will be most frequently evaluated and to test the instrument with individuals who would likely to be using it. It is not likely that the appropriate setting would be a tertiary care university hospital staffed by senior hand surgeons. Again, the specifics of the approach to determine reliability depend on the nature of the instrument and the objectives underlying its development.

Before any validity testing can take place, reliability must be established. It makes no sense to evaluate the validity of the scale if its reliability has not been proven. It will not matter how valid the scale is considered if it cannot be implemented in a reliable fashion. This is a basic tenet of any type of measurement regardless of whether the goal is diagnosis or the evaluation of outcome.

Establishing the validity of a scale should be thought of as a multidimensional activity. There is usually not one approach that ensures the validity of the scale. There may be considerations of content validity, construct validity, convergent or divergent validity, and the need for various types of validity are again dependent on the overall goal.

Essentially validity refers to the idea that the instrument measures reality. In other words, it identifies the phenomenon of interest fully and accurately. In the case of a diagnostic scale, the phenomenon of interest is the presence of a disease state and the objective is to apply the diagnostic label if the condition is identified; because this is what leads to correct decisions regarding treatment and prognosis. Implicit in this concept is the idea that the diagnoses made by the scale can be compared with a known diagnosis because the ability of the instrument to perform effectively in this way is the basis of whether or not it will be considered "valid." However, this implies that there is a way of making the diagnosis definitively without the scale. If there is a way to know definitively that the diagnosis is present, is there a need for a diagnostic scale to begin with? The answer is "yes" if the standard method is difficult, painful, expensive, or in some other way suboptimal. Under these circumstances, if the new scale is shown to demonstrate the same diagnosis without the inconvenience, pain, or expense then it represents an important advance. This introduces the difficult concept of the "gold standard."

WHAT ARE DIAGNOSTIC GOLD STANDARDS?

The term "gold standard" is usually thought of as describing the essential basis for a given process or test. In the area of diagnosis, the gold standard is often considered to be the single criterion that confirms (or less commonly, rules out) a diagnosis.

However, the process of diagnosis is often more complex than this. The role of electrodiagnostic testing in CTS has already been alluded to as an example of a laboratory test that is often used in a way that negates all clinical information because it is considered the gold standard for the diagnosis. In fact, the role that electrodiagnostic tests should occupy in the diagnosis of CTS is not clear and perhaps even controversial,[9] so it would appear that this is not necessarily accepted as a gold standard by all clinicians who diagnose the condition. The key point is that there is no consensus on the matter and where there is no widespread agreement the test cannot be considered to be a gold standard.

To make this point more simplistic it should be considered that an inch is accepted to be 2.54 cm in length. In other words, there is a widely accepted consensus that 2.54 cm is what will constitute an inch; similarly, an ounce will weigh 28.35 grams; and, furthermore, 16 ounces will be something called a pound. The important point is that these are agreed upon measures and as such they form a stable basis on which to move forward with our tasks of measurement.

The idea that there must be consensus to establish a gold standard is not merely pedantic. Where there is agreement there will be reliability—a diagnosis made with agreed upon criterion in one setting is more likely to be made in the same way in a different setting than would be the case where no such consensus exists. This is a consideration that is critical to the acceptance of any diagnostic criterion.

To return to the question of establishing validity, the question of whether a diagnosis made by the instrument is accurate requires comparison to some kind of external standard, and this standard has to be agreed upon by consensus to have meaning. The inherently circular nature of this argument may be troubling to clinicians because of the necessity to have some practical guidelines on which to move forward. It is precisely for this reason that the concept of consensus has to be considered as the basis for making decisions about diagnostic criteria. As knowledge grows, the criteria for making a diagnosis may change and this should be seen as a natural evolution that reflects this increased understanding.

HOW IS CONSENSUS MEASURED?

The ways in which this kind of consensus is established are varied. Usually a relative consensus is implicitly established by what appears in the literature, biased though it may be. This usually reflects the distilled opinions of authors who may or may not be experts on the topic. Consensus can also be actively established through various group processes such as nominal groups, Delphi, and similar activities that seek to bring together experts on the subject for direct or indirect interaction (Graham and colleagues).[8] In fact, the best method of measuring whether consensus exists is also somewhat controversial, but there are certainly stable statistical processes for distinguishing real from spurious agreement among a group.[10] An increased use of these approaches may be dictated by the imperative to seek a basis in evidence for the diagnostic process.

HOW SHOULD DIAGNOSTIC SCALES REPORT THEIR RESULTS?

Regardless of the evidence-based nature of a diagnostic scale, the extent to which clinical users will find it useful to aid the diagnostic process may be largely dependent on the format in which the instrument generates its results. Although the way in which the various diagnostic criteria are assigned importance or combined with each other varies with the condition, most scales invoke some kind of threshold concept to establish the presence of a given diagnosis.

One approach is to assign an ordinal ranking to each of the diagnostic criteria. This is the strategy used by the Jones criteria for the diagnosis of rheumatic fever.[11] Some diagnostic criteria are deemed "major" while others are considered "minor." A critical combination of the various major and minor criteria is used to define the presence of the condition of rheumatic fever.

In this system two minor criteria are considered, for diagnostic purposes, to be equivalent to one major criterion. The idea of making a distinction between major and minor diagnostic criteria appears to appeal to clinicians although the reliability and validity of this approach probably varies substantially with the condition being diagnosed.

An alternative to ordinal ranking is a polythetic threshold. These systems base the diagnosis on the presence of a threshold number of criteria, all of which may be considered to have equal diagnostic significance. The American College of Rheumatology (ACR) criteria for the diagnosis of systemic lupus erythematosis (SLE) is an example of this type of scale.[12] In this system, the diagnosis of SLE is made if any 4 of 11 key clinical or laboratory findings are present. The ACR has developed a similar approach for the diagnosis of rheumatoid arthritis[13] and this strategy is also used for several conditions in the *Diagnostic and Statistical Manual of Mental Disorders IV* (DSM-IV).[14] Like systems that use ordinal rankings, polythetic systems are inherently appealing to clinicians because they may reflect the variable presentation of the conditions they describe. Their main psychometric feature is that reliability is likely to increase with the number of criteria that are considered to have diagnostic importance.

Where the diagnosis has particular importance because of its prognostic implications, or because it may be associated with dangerous or costly treatment, a monothetic strategy may be appropriate. In these systems all of the criteria that are considered to be important have to be met for the diagnosis to be established. This approach does not allow much flexibility, so there are only a few clinical settings in which this may be useful. The DSM-IV uses a monothetic system for some diagnoses.

DIAGNOSIS AS A PROBABILISTIC CONCEPT

Most medical conditions are not diagnosed with the aid of a formalized set of diagnostic criteria that have been rigorously standardized. It is likely that most clinicians actually use a "probabilistic" model in considering whether a given diagnosis is present. In fact, it might be considered that patients do not have a disease but rather a probability of disease.[15] This is really the basis of the process of establishing a differential diagnosis as taught to student clinicians. The list of possible diagnoses to explain a certain clinical presentation is ranked by their individual probabilities of being true. The subsequent steps in the diagnostic process are generally aimed at choosing among these possibilities, usually through re-evaluations and laboratory tests. Eventually this approach culminates in a decision to undertake therapy. Implicit in that decision is the probability that the diagnosis of interest has exceeded a threshold at which therapy is considered safe or advisable. Obviously this threshold may vary dependent on the cost, discomfort, or risk of complications associated with the proposed intervention.[16]

Although such an internalized concept of probability is likely common among diagnosticians, only a few diagnostic scales with this kind of output have been developed.[5,17,18] In general, the need to invoke treatment as a result of diagnosis may suggest a need to be more definitive than a probabilistic approach implies. In addition, describing the diagnosis in probabilistic terms may be confusing or even distressing for some patients, even where it may represent a more accurate description of their condition than a definitive statement implying that the diagnosis is certain.

On the other hand a probabilistic approach to diagnosis has a few clear advantages. First, there is frequently some uncertainty associated with diagnosis. The capacity to quantify that uncertainty in probabilistic terms could actually be helpful in discussing prognosis and treatment with patients. Second, having knowledge of the probability of a diagnosis may help define whether additional testing is required if the need for this testing is defined in terms of the increase (or decrease) in the probability of the diagnosis. In a climate of cost containment, the value of diagnostic testing may be better understood using these Bayesian concepts. A third advantage is that thinking of diagnosis in probabilistic terms allows clinicians a certain degree of flexibility in linking diagnosis to treatment. For example, for conditions like CTS, which may occur in a workplace setting, the threshold, in diagnostic probability terms, for advising surgical treatment may differ if the diagnosis is made in the context of a workers' compensation claim.

WHERE DO WE GO FROM HERE?

To summarize, a critical issue for clinicians to acknowledge is the need for accurate, reliable diagnostic criteria for the conditions they evaluate because this the basis for rational, effective treatment and the estimation of a meaningful prognosis. Standardizing diagnostic approaches wherever this is feasible can reduce variations in care. The development of diagnostic scales has the potential to meet this goal, just as the creation of outcome measures has made the evaluation of the outcome of care more uniform. The approaches to the development of diagnostic scales should follow the same measurement principles used in the development of outcome instruments. The concept of consensus is fundamental to understanding how we make diagnoses and should be thought of as a potentially flexible and fluid idea that can accommodate the discovery of new knowledge in our efforts to accurately diagnose medical conditions.

REFERENCES

1. Eddy DM, Clanton CH. The art of diagnosis: solving the clinicopathological exercise. N Engl J Med 1982; 306(21):1263–8.
2. Berner ES, Miller RA, Graber ML. Missed and delayed diagnoses in the ambulatory setting. Ann Intern Med 2007;146(6):470 [author reply 470–1].
3. Ladouceur M, Rahme E, Pineau CA, et al. Robustness of prevalence estimates derived from misclassified data from administrative databases. Biometrics 2007;63(1):272–9.
4. Graham B, Dvali L, Regehr G, et al. Variations in diagnostic criteria for carpal tunnel syndrome among Ontario specialists. Am J Ind Med 2006;49(1):8–13.

5. Graham B, et al. Development and validation of diagnostic criteria for carpal tunnel syndrome. J Hand Surg [Am] 2006;31(6):919–24.

6. Sackett D, Haynes RB, Guyatt GH, et al. Clinical epidemiology, a basic science for clinical medicine. 2nd edition. Toronto: Little, Brown; 1991.

7. Streiner D, Norman GR. Health measurement scales, a practical guide to their development and use. 2nd edition. Oxford (UK): Oxford University Press; 1995.

8. Graham B, Regehr G, Wright JG. Delphi as a method to establish consensus for diagnostic criteria. J Clin Epidemiol 2003;56(12):1150–6.

9. Graham B. The value added of electrodiagnostic testing in the diagnosis of carpal tunnel syndrome. J Bone Joint Surg, in press.

10. Gustafson D, Fryback DG, Rose JH, et al. A decision theoretic methodology for severity index development. Med Decis Making 1986;6(1):27–35.

11. Special writing group of the Committee on Rheumatic Fever, Endocarditis, and Kawasaki disease of the Council on Cardiovascular Disease in the Young of the American Heart Association. Guidelines for the diagnosis of rheumatic fever. Jones criteria, 1992 update. JAMA 1992;268(15):2069–73.

12. Hochberg MC. Updating the American College of Rheumatology revised criteria for the classification of systemic lupus erythematosus. Arthritis Rheum 1997;40(9):1725.

13. Arnett FC, Edworthy SM, Bloch DA, et al. The American Rheumatism Association 1987 revised criteria for classification of rheumatoid arthritis. Arthritis Rheum 1988;31(3):315–24.

14. Special writing group of the Committee on Rheumatic Fever, Endocarditis, and Kawasaki disease of the Council on Cardiovascular Disease in the Young of the American Heart Association. Diagnostic and statistical manual of mental disorders: DSM-IV. 4th edition. Washington, DC: American Psychiatric Association; 1994.

15. Sheps SB, Schechter MT. The assessment of diagnostic tests. A survey of current medical research. JAMA 1984;252(17):2418–22.

16. Kaplan RM, Ganiats TG, Frosch DL. Diagnostic and treatment decisions in US healthcare. J Health Psychol 2004;9(1):29–40.

17. Wigton RS, Hoellerich VL, Ornato JP, et al. Use of clinical findings in the diagnosis of urinary tract infection in women. Arch Intern Med 1985;145(12):2222–7.

18. Poses RM, Cebul RD, Collins M, et al. The importance of disease prevalence in transporting clinical prediction rules. The case of streptococcal pharyngitis. Ann Intern Med 1986;105(4):586–91.

Using Evidence-Based Practice to Select Diagnostic Tests

Jean-Sébastien Roy, PT, PhD(c)[a],*,
Susan Michlovitz, PhD, PT, CHT[b,c]

KEYWORDS

- Evidence-based medicine
- Carpal tunnel syndrome • Diagnostic tests
- Hand • Sensitivity and specificity

Diagnosis is a primary activity of hand surgeons and therapists that is fundamental in the definition of appropriate clinical questions for evidence-based practice (EBP). Sound diagnostic tests can be used to assist in "ruling in" or "ruling out" a condition to best direct prognosis and treatment. It is apparent from the collective experiences of hand care professionals that the assigning of the diagnostic label is not always obvious. This can present a dilemma for the clinician; if you make an incorrect diagnosis it is unlikely the treatment will be successful. Therefore, to be able to execute good clinical decision making, your diagnostic decisions must be made using the most accurate diagnostic tests along with logical and solid clinical judgment. The purpose of this article is to demonstrate how EBP can help improve the diagnostic process by using the five steps to assist in selecting the best diagnostic tests with known accuracy and sound test properties.[1]

HOW TO START THE EVIDENCE-BASED PRACTICE PROCESS

If you review the history and description of symptoms in the example case (**Box 1**), your clinical experience would be used to develop an overall impression (sometimes called a pretest probability). Your past clinical experience and information provided by this patient might suggest that this woman has carpal tunnel syndrome (CTS). First, she reports waking up at night with numb hands, a symptom that is common in patients with CTS. Second, she is a jeweler; therefore, she has relevant work exposure because she has to perform repetitive grasping and manipulative activities sometimes in the wrist flexed position. Third, although she has not been specific with the location of her numbness, it is common for patients with CTS initially on interview to be vague about the location of their pain and numbness within the hand. Fourth, the peak prevalence of CTS is among women aged 55 years and older.[2]

That being considered, there are some elements in her history that could suggest that she might have a different or concurrent disorder. She has occasional neck pain; therefore, her forearm pain and hand numbness could originate from a cervical radiculopathy. Her forearm pain could also be suggestive of tendinosis. Finally, Heberden's nodes are most likely associated with osteoarthritis. Because it is not uncommon to see osteoarthritis in patients with CTS, this could be a comorbid problem. Based on your clinical experience, you define the pretest probability of the different potential diagnoses. Hand care professionals may use a subjective evaluation to estimate the pretest probability by using their personal experience with similar patients and by knowing the frequency of the potential disease in those patients. Therefore,

---

[a] School of Rehabilitation Science, McMaster University, Hamilton, Ontario L8S 1C7, Canada
[b] Cayuga Hand Therapy Physical Therapy, 15 Lisa Lane, Ithaca, NY, USA
[c] Rehabilitation Medicine, Columbia University, NY, USA
* Corresponding author.
E-mail address: jean-sebastien.roy.1@ulaval.ca (J-S. Roy)

Hand Clin 25 (2009) 49–57
doi:10.1016/j.hcl.2008.09.004

Box 1
Case example

A 58-year-old female jeweler comes into your office complaining of tingling in both hands and pain in the forearms with the right worst than the left. She wakes at night with numb hands. On examination you note she has Heberden's nodes on the dorsum of the distal phalanges. She also reports occasional pain in her neck. She denies having diabetes or hypothyroidism.

---

you conclude by best guess that the most probable diagnosis (say 75% probability) for this patient is CTS. Alternative diagnoses that might explain the patient's symptoms include neck radiculopathy (35% probability), tendinosis (20% probability), and osteoarthritis (10% probability). At this point, you need to select diagnostic tests that are based on best evidence to help you increase your confidence in a definitive diagnosis. You would like the most specific test available to confirm (rule in) CTS and the most sensitive test to establish that CTS is unlikely (rule out). How can you find and select clinical diagnostic tests with these properties?

We should select tests that have been tested and have been shown to have diagnostic accuracy (the ability to discriminate accurately between patients with and without a specific disorder or condition in question) and reliability (produces precise, accurate, and reproducible information) in high-quality studies. The contemporary medical literature is abundant in articles where researchers have assessed the diagnostic utility of tests. Diagnostic accuracy is often expressed in terms of positive and negative predictive values, sensitivity and specificity, and likelihood ratios (**Table 1**). By using principles of EBP (including clinical expertise) to select the best diagnostic tests and applying the best information on what accuracy they will have in our clinical situation, we can make more definitive diagnoses and be better able to guide treatment.

Principles of EBP may help hand therapists and surgeons become more evidence-based in their application of diagnostic tests. EBP can be defined in terms of five steps that serve to structure decision making and ensure optimum use of clinicians' expertise in the diagnosis (**Table 2**).[1] Clinicians not only need to be able to identify the best evidence to address the patient's concern, but also must use their expertise to interpret the evidence and apply it appropriately to their patient's situation.[3] We will use the case example

described earlier to illustrate how the five steps are used to select diagnostic tests for CTS.

THE FIVE STEPS OF EVIDENCE-BASED PRACTICE
Ask a Specific Clinical Question

The first step in using EBP to select diagnostic tests is to decide what information you need about the patient. You can begin by formulating a good clinical question. Therefore you want to translate your uncertainty about a definitive diagnosis to formulate a relevant, answerable clinical question that will facilitate your literature search.[1] You have to decide what details are important for making a diagnosis to find the best evidence available.[3]

Clinicians must choose tests that will be the most helpful in the diagnostic decision-making process. In the case of a patient with CTS, a variety of diagnostic tests have been described.[4–8] These tests range from (1) tests focusing on the nature of the symptoms, like Katz's hand symptom diagram, subjective complaints of swelling, and nocturnal paresthesia; (2) provocative tests, like Phalen's maneuver, reverse Phalen's, Durkan's carpal compression, Tinel's test, tourniquet Gilliat, diagnostic ultrasound, tethered median nerve stress, and lumbrical provocation; (3) sensory/motor tests, like touch threshold with Semmes-Weinstein monofilaments, vibration threshold, current perception threshold, two-point discrimination, thenar weakness and thenar atrophy; or (4) electrodiagnostic tests. As you can see, many diagnostic tests are available for CTS. But are they accurate (both sensitive and specific)? Have they been evaluated for their validity and reliability? Which ones should you use in your practice to "rule in" or "rule out" CTS? To conduct all the described diagnostic tests on each patient would be an inefficient use of time and resources and a waste of the patient's time. You would probably find divergence in their results.[4] Therefore, you have to decide, based on best evidence, which tests and maneuvers to use in your clinical practice when dealing with a patient whose symptoms are consistent with what you suspect is CTS.

Back to the case example: In the past you may have used clinical tests to help you with the diagnosis of patients with signs and symptoms related to CTS. However, you may never have searched for the properties of these clinical diagnostic tests. Therefore, you have established a clinical question: *"Which clinical diagnostic tests have the highest level of sensitivity and specificity to establish if a 58-year-old woman with symptoms of CTS actually has this syndrome?"*

Table 1
Utility of diagnostic tests: operational definitions

	Definition	Formula to Calculate	Interpretation of Findings
Positive predictive values	Used to predict that a patient DOES have a condition	True positive/(true positive + false positive)	How well a positive test result correctly predicts the presence of the disease or condition
Negative predictive value	Used to predict that a patient does NOT have a condition	True negative/(false negative + true negative)	How well a negative test result correctly predicts the absence of the disease or condition
Sensitivity	Can detect when a patient DOES has a condition	True positive/(true positive + false negative)	The test can be used to "rule out" a diagnosis; ie, if most cases are detected then a negative test rules out
Specificity	Can detect when a patient does NOT have a condition	True negative/(false positive + true negative)	The test can be done to "rule in" a diagnosis; ie, if most normality is detected then a positive test rules in
Positive likelihood ratio	Can predict likelihood of someone HAVING a disorder if the diagnostic test result(s) is (are) positive	Sensitivity/(1-specificity)	The best test to use for "ruling in" the disease or condition is the one with the largest likelihood ratio of a positive test
Negative likelihood ratio	Can predict likelihood of someone NOT having a disorder if the diagnostic test result(s) is (are) negative	(1-sensitivity)/specificity	The best test to use for "ruling out" the disease or condition is the one with the smaller likelihood ratio of a negative test

Your question could have been more specific to a clinical diagnostic test that you usually used, such as: *"When compared with electrodiagnosis tests, what are the sensitivity and specificity of the Tinel's test to determine if a 58-year-old woman with symptoms of CTS actually has this syndrome."* In this last example, we find the four components usually found in a well-built clinical question, which are (1) patient or problems, (2) diagnostic test under review, (3) comparison diagnostic test (gold-standard), and (4) outcome.[1]

Find the Best Evidence to Answer the Question

Once the clinical question is formulated, you need to track down evidence to answer your question. When possible, your search should try to target the highest possible levels of evidence, eg, Levels 1 and 2. However, the question posed may or may not have a reasonable and appropriate range of research and evidence available in the literature on testing for your clinically suspected condition(s).

The best levels of evidence for diagnostic tests are found, according to the Oxford Center for Evidence-based Medicine (www.cebm.net), in the following:

Level 1a
- Systematic reviews of level 1 diagnostic studies (prospective cohorts, blind and independent comparison to high-quality gold standard diagnoses)
- Clinical decision rule (scoring systems that lead to a diagnostic category) with 1b studies from different clinical centers

Table 2
The five steps of EBP to select diagnostic tests

The Five Steps	Examples to Select Diagnostic Tests for Carpal Tunnel Syndrome
1. Ask a specific clinical question	Which diagnostic tests have the highest level of sensitivity and specificity to establish if a 58-year-old woman with symptoms of CTS actually has this syndrome?
2. Find the best evidence to answer the question	Using keywords such as "carpal tunnel syndrome," "diagnosis," "sensitivity" or "specificity," you perform a search in Medline to find the best levels of evidence for CTS diagnostic tests.
3. Critically appraise the evidence for its validity and usefulness	You critically appraise the evidence to choose accurate tests that are valid, reliable, and applicable to your population and clinical setting.
4. Integrate appraisal results with clinical expertise and patient values	You integrate the best evidence to your clinical setting. Therefore, you choose three diagnostic tests that are either highly specific or sensible, or both: (1) Katz hand diagram, (2) carpal compression combined with wrist flexion test, and, (3) static two-point test.
5. Evaluate the outcomes	You evaluate if outcome measurements demonstrate the impact of your clinical decisions. You use a self-reported questionnaire, the DASH and CTSQ, to measure the symptoms of your patients following the intervention chosen according to the results of CTS diagnostic tests.

Level 1b
- Validating cohort study with good reference standards
- Clinical decision rule tested within one clinical center

Level 1c
- Study with a diagnostic finding whose specificity is so high that a positive test rules-in the diagnosis
- Study with sensitivity so high that a negative result rules-out the diagnosis.

It is important to develop efficient search strategies when looking for the best available evidence in the literature. Using one or more keywords, a structured search can be conducted. For our case example, keywords such as "carpal tunnel syndrome," "diagnosis," "sensitivity," or "specificity" can be combined in the search strategy to find diagnostic tests for CTS. In a systematic review on clinical diagnostic tests for CTS, 1015 abstracts were found when performing a search in Medline and CINAHL using a combination of these four keywords.[4] After reviewing the abstract, the authors found that only 75 articles of the 1015 really addressed the diagnostic accuracy of clinical diagnostic tests for CTS.[4] This illustrates the

need for efficient searches and the values of a systematic review.

The quality of the studies found when performing such a search is variable. Therefore, the hand care professionals have to critically appraise the evidence found in the studies to evaluate the validity and usefulness of the clinical diagnostic tests proposed. Since most of the hand care professionals do not usually have the time to critically appraise, for example, 75 articles before choosing the right diagnostic tools, they often rely on systematic reviews and meta-analysis. For CTS, systematic reviews have been published that will help the clinicians in their search for diagnostic tests.[4,9,10]

Critically Appraise the Evidence For Its Validity and Usefulness

If you are fortunate enough to find a systematic review on a diagnostic test (this rarely occurs), you may find that DARE (Database of Abstracts of Reviews of Effects) has performed a critical appraisal. DARE is a database that systematically identifies and assesses the quality of systematic reviews (www.crd.york.ac.uk/crdweb). If DARE has performed a critical appraisal, then the following methodological criteria will be addressed: (1) Were inclusion/exclusion criteria reported? (2) Was the search adequate? (3) Were the included studies synthesized? (4) Was the validity of the included studies assessed? (5) Are sufficient details about the individual included studies presented? These criteria can also be useful to the hand care professionals if they wish to critically appraise systematic reviews.

If you choose to critically appraise studies from a primary source (original data), then there are certain aspects that you need to verify. The questions you should ask when applying a diagnostic study to your practice include the following:

- What was the setting for the study?
- Are the results valid and reliable?
- Is there a consensus on the gold standard?
- Was the gold standard applied to all cases?
- Did the sample include an appropriate spectrum of patients similar to those found in the general practice?
- Are the findings clinically relevant to your population and clinical setting?
- Is the test described with enough details to be replicated in your clinical setting?
- Were there blind evaluators?
- What is the rational of the test?
- What is a normal response?

You will try to answer these questions with the critical appraisal that you perform. It will help in your decision to choose accurate tests that are valid, reliable and applicable to your population and clinical setting. This is a necessary step to ensure that the changes that you will be making in your practice are not based on invalid and unreliable research or on untested ideas that were handed down over time. To understand how to critically appraise diagnostic tests, we will follow guidelines proposed by Sackett and colleagues.[1]

Accuracy

To establish diagnosis accuracy, a diagnostic test has first to be compared with an accepted reference standard, often referred to as a "gold standard."[11] For pathology such as CTS, there is a lack of agreement on an accepted "gold standard."[4] Positive responses to carpal tunnel release, injection, electrodiagnosis, and expert clinical diagnosis have been proposed as potential "gold standard" diagnoses.[4] However, there is no consensus on these proposed "gold standards,"[4,12] and, presently, electrodiagnosis tests are the most widely used comparators in studies evaluating CTS diagnostic tests.[4,13]

For example, some investigators have decided to evaluate the properties of the Tinel's test in the diagnosis of the CTS. As the gold standard, they have chosen electrodiagnostic tests. Therefore, results from Tinel's test (diagnostic test under review) are compared with blinded results from electrodiagnostic tests (gold standard) using a two-by-two table (**Table 3**). From this table, the positive and negative predictive values, sensitivity, specificity, and likelihood ratios of the diagnostic test under review can be estimated (see **Table 1**).

A systematic review has estimated the sensitivity and specificity of the Tinel's test by averaging values across studies weighted by sample size.[4] They have observed that the average sensitivity is 50, and the average specificity is 77. Therefore, 50% of the patients that had been identified by the gold standard as having CTS were correctly identified by the Tinel's test (sensitivity: proportion of actual positives that are correctly identified as such); whereas, 77% of the patients who did not present CTS when evaluated by the gold standard were correctly identified as not having CTS by the Tinel's test (specificity: percentage of well people who are identified as not having the condition). According to this systematic review,[4] the three clinical diagnostic tests with the highest sensitivity for CTS are carpal compression combined with wrist flexion and current perception threshold (80%) followed by Katz hand diagram (75%); and with the highest specificity are static two-point (95%), Thenar atrophy (94%), and carpal compression combined with wrist flexion (92%). Hand surgeons and therapists must be aware that no single test ensures a correct diagnosis and that all tests are subject to errors.[5]

Table 3
Two-by-two table

		Gold standard	
		Patient HAS CTS	Patient does NOT have CTS
Diagnostic test under review	Patient appears to HAVE CTS	True positive	False positive
	Patient appears NOT to have CTS	False negative	True negative

Once these psychometric properties are known, the clinician can decide which clinical diagnostic tests have the quality required to be used as diagnosing tools for CTS. The tests under review should have something new to offer compared with the gold standard; otherwise, there is no reason to choose another test than the gold standard. For example, the carpal compression combined with wrist flexion test is less costly and less risky, clearly more comfortable, and quicker to perform than electrodiagnostic tests.

When critically appraising a study, you have to verify if the investigators have evaluated a sample of patients that include an appropriate spectrum of patients (ie, a spectrum that is similar to those found in the general practice). Therefore, the diagnostic tests have to be evaluated on a sample that includes patients with mild, moderate, and severe CTS. Furthermore, the control group in the study should not be composed of healthy subjects. Investigators should recruit a population that is similar to what is seen in the clinical setting. The diagnostic challenge is not replicated when using subjects who do not have any hand symptoms. Therefore, proper research design necessitates that the noncases (patients who do not have CTS) should have either compression neuropathy in a different area or different pathologies that affect the wrist or hand.[5] In fact, it has been shown that studies using healthy controls report higher specificity than those that use control patients with wrist symptoms, but negative electrodiagnostic test results.[4] For example, the specificity of the Tinel's test when healthy subjects are used as controls is 84%, whereas it drops to 65% when the control group is composed of patients presenting wrist symptoms with negative electrodiagnostic tests.[4,7] In the case of CTS, this reflects problems with electrodiagnostic tests as the gold standard and increased difficulty in discrimination when presented with actual patients with symptoms that overlap competing diagnoses.

The use of a blinded evaluator is also essential. If the same examiner performs the gold standard evaluation (for example, electrodiagnostic tests) as well as the diagnostic test under review (for example, the Tinel's test), there is a risk of bias, especially if the examiner is biased toward a particular test. Therefore, different evaluators should perform the two tests, and the evaluator applying and interpreting the diagnostic tests under review should not be aware of the results obtained with the gold standard.

Reliability

The reliability of the diagnostic tests should also be shown. Therefore, the results obtained by a diagnostic test must be reproducible by the same clinician in time or be two different evaluators if the condition of the patients is unchanged. Moreover, the challenge of showing that a diagnostic test is reliable increases when expertise is required in performing and interpreting the test. For example, investigators have evaluated the intra- and interobserver reliability of the touch threshold (Semmes-Weinstein monofilament) test, and Tinel's and Phalen's tests on 12 subjects with possible CTS.[14] For these three tests, the intraobserver was good, with intraclass correlation coefficient (ICC) of 0.71 for touch threshold, and kappa of 0.77 and 0.65 for Tinel's and Phalen's tests. In contrast, the interobserver reliability was poor for touch threshold (ICC = 0.15), whereas it was moderate to good for Tinel's ($\kappa = 0.80$) and Phalen's ($\kappa = 0.53$) tests. The touch threshold is a diagnostic test with more variation in application techniques and decision rules, which is reflected in the interobserver reliability.

Performing and interpreting tests

Once you have found a diagnostic test that has been shown to be reliable and valid, you have to know how to use it. Hand care professionals need to know how to perform the diagnostic tests and interpret the results, as well as the requirements, standardization, and equipment needed. If you are using provocative, sensory, or motor tests: What is the pressure that you should use? What kind of symptoms should you elicit (pain or tingling)? What precautions should be taken during and after the test? You need to know the reasons explaining a positive or a negative test result (the rationale of the test) and what a normal/abnormal response to a test should be. For example, the rationale for the Tinel's test is that regenerative nerve fibers are susceptible to mechanical deformation. The method that has been described to perform the Tinel's test is for the examiner to tap with fingertips along the median nerve at the carpal tunnel.[15] The positive result shows tingling or electric shocks felt along the median nerve.[15]

Finally, the investigators have to show the utility of the tests, that is, that the test will help you in the diagnosis of your patients and will get you beyond the point that you were before performing it. Furthermore, the risks of performing the test, if there is risk, should not go beyond the benefits that the results could bring. You must make sure the test will really be valuable in detecting the problem and then leading to treatment to improve the well-being of your patients.

Integrate Appraisal Results with Clinical Expertise and Patient Goals/Values

The fourth step is the integration of the best evidence to your clinical setting. Once you have determined which diagnostic tests are accurate, as well as relevant and applicable for your patients, you have to apply this evidence in your clinical practice. Therefore, you need to implement the appropriate findings and recommendations. This is the process of change management and a series of clinical decisions have to be taken. You have to identify the important recommendations, and whether these recommendations are applicable to your patient. You also have to look to see if there are any risks for adverse effects and if so, how you can avoid them. All evidence should be integrated with clinical expertise, patient preference, and values in making a practice decision and change.

You will have to determine what specific skills will be needed to perform and interpret the diagnostic tests and what will be the specific implementation sequence of these tests. Tests should be affordable and available in your clinical setting or easily accessible. For a test like the Tinel's, this is not an issue because no equipment is needed. For a test like the touch threshold, which requires equipment and clinical expertise, you must decide if the expense is worth the benefits or if cheaper alternatives would suffice. Hand surgeons and therapists also have to determine if the use of the diagnostic tests will affect their management of CTS and how the evidence will influence their choice of treatment. Thereafter, once your selected changes have been implemented in your clinical setting, you will need to observe the effects of your diagnostic decisions on the patient outcomes.

Back to the case example: You have decided, based on clinical experience, literature search, and critical appraisal, to perform three clinical diagnostic tests to evaluate your patient. You have chosen (1) the Katz hand diagram because it is a subjective test with high sensitivity, (2) the carpal compression combined with wrist flexion test because it is a provocative test with high sensitivity and specificity, and (3) the static two-point test because it is a sensory test with high specificity. Moreover, you have used these three tests in the past, therefore you have the clinical expertise required to perform and interpret these tests. You perform these three tests and the three have positive results for CTS. You also chose to perform a diagnostic test to rule out cervical radiculopathy. You perform the neck distraction test because it is highly specific (0.90) for cervical radiculopathy.[16] The neck distraction test turns out to be negative. Therefore, based on your clinical experience and because you have used accurate clinical diagnostic tests (with either high specificity or sensitivity, or both), you are now more confident about the diagnosis of your patient and you can move on to choose the proper intervention (**Table 4**). The posttest probability for CTS (clinical predictive rules)[17] when these three CTS diagnostic tests are used has not been evaluated. However, it has been shown that positive results of the following five variables were associated with a posttest probability for CTS of 90%: (1) symptoms improve with moving, "shaking" or positioning the wrist or hand, (2) wrist-ratio index greater than 0.67, (3) Brigham and Women's Hospital Hand Symptom Severity Scale score greater than 1.9, (4) diminished sensation in median sensory field 1 (thumb), and (5) age greater than 45 years.[13]

Evaluate the Outcomes

The last step in this process is to evaluate the effectiveness and efficacy of your decisions in direct relation to your patients. You have to validate that your diagnoses were improved when using

Table 4
How accurate diagnostic tests results affect your confidence

Potential Diagnosis	Pre-Test Probability	Diagnostic tests performed		Post-Tests Confidence Over the Diagnosis
		Diagnostic Tests	Result	
Carpal tunnel syndrome	75%	Katz hand diagram	+	Increased
		Carpal compression combined with wrist flexion test	+	
		Static two-point test	+	
Cervical radiculopathy	35%	Neck distraction test	−	Decreased
Tendinosis	20%			Decreased
Osteoarthritis	10%			Decreased

accurate diagnostic tests based on your literature search and on your critical appraisal of the literature. Therefore, you should evaluate if outcome measurements demonstrate the impact on your patients. Such measures may be physiologic (complication reduction, health improvement), psychosocial (quality of life, patient perception of care), or functional improvement. You also need to interpret the results considering the apparent severity of nerve compression, potential confounding conditions, and physical and psychosocial factors.[5] It could be expected that if the diagnosis is correct then this patient with proper treatment would experience a reduction in symptom severity as measured by the Boston Carpal Tunnel Symptom Severity Scale.[18]

You can check regularly to see if there is new information in the literature on the diagnostic tests for the CTS and see how you can improve and update your clinical decisions. All of these elements require thoughtful action and keeping up-to-date with the current literature.

Back to the case example. Following your diagnosis, you ask another clinical question: What is the effectiveness of conservative interventions in the management of CTS? Again, you performed a review and critical appraisal of the literature related to the conservative interventions for CTS. Your conclusions are that you should start your intervention with full-time splinting.[19,20] Before starting your intervention, your patient completes two established self-reported questionnaires: the Brigham and Woman's Hospital Carpal Tunnel Specific Questionnaire (CTSQ) and the Disabilities of the Arm, Shoulder, and Hand (DASH). Four weeks after the beginning of the intervention, your patient is reevaluated. She says that her symptom severity has decreased (60% less pain and no hand numbness during the night). You also note that there is a significant improvement in the CTSQ and DASH scores. Therefore, accurate diagnostic tests combined with logical and solid clinical judgment have helped to efficiently guide your intervention, and ultimately improve the symptoms of your patient.

SUMMARY

Hand care professionals need to understand the principles of evidence-based practice (EBP) to base clinical decisions on the best available evidence. We have illustrated how the five steps of EBM guide us to select high-quality evidence for diagnostic tests. Hand surgeons or therapists can use this process combined with their clinical expertise to perform optimal EBP-supported clinical decision making.

REFERENCES

1. Sackett DL, Straus SE, Richardson WS, et al. Evidence-based medicine: how to practice and teach EBM. 3rd edition. Edinburgh, UK: Churchill Livingstone; 2005.
2. Atroshi I, Gummesson C, Johnsson R, et al. Prevalence of carpal tunnel syndrome in a general population. JAMA 1999;282(2):153–8.
3. Cleland JA, Noteboom JT, Whitman JM, et al. A primer on selected aspects of evidence-based practice relating to questions of treatment, part 1: asking questions, finding evidence, and determining validity. J Orthop Sports Phys Ther 2008;38(8):476–84.
4. MacDermid JC, Wessel J. Clinical diagnosis of carpal tunnel syndrome: a systematic review. J Hand Ther 2004;17(2):309–19.
5. MacDermid JC, Doherty T. Clinical and electrodiagnostic testing of carpal tunnel syndrome: a narrative review. J Orthop Sports Phys Ther 2004;34(10):565–88.
6. Ghavanini MR, Haghighat M. Carpal tunnel syndrome: reappraisal of five clinical tests. Electromyogr Clin Neurophysiol 1998;38(7):437–41.
7. Szabo RM, Slater RR Jr, Farver TB, et al. The value of diagnostic testing in carpal tunnel syndrome. J Hand Surg [Am] 1999;24(4):704–14.
8. de Krom MC, Knipschild PG, Kester AD, et al. Efficacy of provocative tests for diagnosis of carpal tunnel syndrome. Lancet 1990;335(8686):393–5.
9. Massy-Westropp N, Grimmer K, Bain G. A systematic review of the clinical diagnostic tests for carpal tunnel syndrome. J Hand Surg [Am] 2000;25(1):120–7.
10. D'Arcy CA, McGee S. The rational clinical examination. Does this patient have carpal tunnel syndrome? JAMA 2000;283(23):3110–7.
11. Fritz JM, Wainner RS. Examining diagnostic tests: an evidence-based perspective. Phys Ther 2001;81(9):1546–64.
12. Kaymak B, Ozcakar L, Cetin A, et al. A comparison of the benefits of sonography and electrophysiologic measurements as predictors of symptom severity and functional status in patients with carpal tunnel syndrome. Arch Phys Med Rehabil 2008;89(4):743–8.
13. Wainner RS, Fritz JM, Irrgang JJ, et al. Development of a clinical prediction rule for the diagnosis of carpal tunnel syndrome. Arch Phys Med Rehabil 2005;86(4):609–18.
14. Marx RG, Hudak PL, Bombardier C, et al. The reliability of physical examination for carpal tunnel syndrome. J Hand Surg [Br] 1998;23(4):499–502.
15. Alfonso MI, Dzwierzynski W. Hoffman-Tinel sign. The realities. Phys Med Rehabil Clin N Am 1998;9(4):721–36.

16. Wainner RS, Fritz JM, Irrgang JJ, et al. Reliability and diagnostic accuracy of the clinical examination and patient self-report measures for cervical radiculopathy. Spine 2003;28(1):52–62.

17. Childs JD, Cleland JA. Development and application of clinical prediction rules to improve decision making in physical therapist practice. Phys Ther 2006; 86(1):122–31.

18. Levine DW, Simmons BP, Koris MJ, et al. A self-administered questionnaire for the assessment of severity of symptoms and functional status in carpal tunnel syndrome. J Bone Joint Surg [Am] 1993; 75(11):1585–92.

19. Muller M, Tsui D, Schnurr R, et al. Effectiveness of hand therapy interventions in primary management of carpal tunnel syndrome: a systematic review. J Hand Ther 2004;17(2):210–28.

20. Hentz VR, Lalonde DH. MOC-PS(SM) CME article: self-assessment and performance in practice: the carpal tunnel. Plast Reconstr Surg 2008;121(4):1–10.

Making Decisions About Prognosis in Evidence-Based Practice

Ryan M. Degen, BSc[a], Daniel J. Hoppe, BSc[a],
Bradley A. Petrisor, MD, MSc, FRCSC[b],*,
Mohit Bhandari, MD, MSc, FRCSC[b]

KEYWORDS

- Evidence-based medicine • Prognosis
- Decision-making • Distal radius

PURPOSE

Evidence-based practice, incorporating the principles stressed in evidence-based medicine,[1,2] includes acquiring and applying the best available evidence and integrating this evidence with the physician's clinical expertise and patient values and preferences to establish a treatment. This approach places less emphasis on expert opinion and nonsystematic clinical observations and, instead, stresses the importance of using evidence derived from clinical research, including randomized-controlled trials and observational studies. Physicians need to be aware of published results that may have an impact on their own practice. For this reason, when faced with a question whose answer is not known, surgeons or physicians may find it useful to examine the literature to identify those results that may apply to their patients. The purpose of this article is to illustrate how a surgeon would find answers to questions on prognosis, using a clinical scenario involving a patient with a distal radius fracture, and then apply what was learned to his or her own practice.

SCENARIO

You are a consulting surgeon asked to see a 67-year-old man referred to you by a local emergency room (ER) physician and who suffered a comminuted distal radius fracture after slipping in his bathtub. The current injury was reduced and splinted; however, the reduction was unstable and will need surgical intervention for more definitive management.

On examining the patient, you find an elderly man who appears in good health. Aside from the current injury, he is otherwise healthy with no comorbidities or other injuries from the fall. After removing the cast you examine his dominant, right wrist and determine that it is neurovascularly intact but with an obvious, closed deformity of the distal radius. There is significant dorsal displacement, confirmed on anteroposterior (AP) and lateral radiographs.

Given your patient's independent lifestyle, you recognize that nonoperative management will not sufficiently restore his level of function,[3] and that he is at risk for secondary displacement with a closed reduction.[4] In terms of operative management, you are also aware that volar locking plates are favored over dorsal plates in internal fixation of distal radius fractures, as there are fewer incidences of extensor tendon irritation after plate application.[3,5,6] For these reasons, you decide your patient would benefit most from open reduction and internal fixation using a volar locking plate.

As you discuss the procedure with the patient, he interjects with a few questions, mentioning that the emergency physician described his break

---

[a] Division of Orthopedic Surgery, Michael G. DeGroote School of Medicine, McMaster University, 2100 Main Street W, Hamilton, Ontario L8N 3Z5, Canada
[b] Division of Orthopaedic Surgery, Department of Surgery, McMaster University, 6N, Hamilton Health Sciences, General Hospital, 237 Barton Street East, Hamilton, Ontario L8L 2X2, Canada
* Corresponding author.
E-mail address: petrisor@hhsc.ca (B.A. Petrisor).

Hand Clin 25 (2009) 59–66
doi:10.1016/j.hcl.2008.09.005
0749-0712/08/$ – see front matter © 2009 Elsevier Inc. All rights reserved.

as "complex," and he worries that the perceived severity of the break at his age will reduce the chances of a successful outcome of the procedure. Because he is also an avid tennis player, he is concerned about diminished functionality given that the break occurred in his dominant hand. You therefore arrange a preop visit at your office the next day to allow yourself time to consult the literature and address his concerns.

LITERATURE SEARCH

Later that evening, you consult the literature to find an article that provides prognostic information on volar plating of distal radius fractures. Your search must be sufficiently broad enough to include all relevant articles, yet focused to be applicable to your patient.

PubMed (www.ncbi.nlm.nih.gov/PubMed) is your starting point, as you are most familiar with this database. You could also consult other databases such as the World of Science and EMBASE. In PubMed, the search terms "distal radius AND (outcomes OR predictors) AND internal fixation" generates 44 results: a feasible number of articles to work through.

A scan of titles and quick read of abstracts identifies two potential studies: "Predictors of Functional Outcomes After Surgical Treatment of Distal Radius Fractures"[7] and "Functional Outcome and Complications After Volar Plating for Dorsally Displaced, Unstable Fractures of the Distal Radius."[8]

WHAT IS A PROGNOSTIC STUDY?

In order for a surgeon to provide care to a patient and offer information about the likelihood of a successful outcome following surgery, he must be aware of variables that accurately predict when patients will do well. These are known as prognostic factors.[9]

For example, in a patient suffering from moderate, but not incapacitating, carpal tunnel syndrome, one option may be a surgical release. According to Radwin and colleagues,[10] patients who demonstrate some level of symptomatic relief with steroid injection show increased success rates with surgical carpal tunnel release.[10] The response to steroid injection can be considered a prognostic variable that correlates positively with improved postoperative pain relief. As a result, the surgeon may first try steroids preoperatively to confirm his decision to recommend surgery. The additional knowledge of prognostic factors facilitates identification of candidates who will benefit

from surgery and improves the surgeon's clinical decision making.

Prognostic studies examine prognostic variables to determine their relationship to disease and its treatment and attempts to predict the probability associated with their effect.[11] If the studies are well conducted, they will distinguish subgroups of patients based on prognostic variables such as gender, age, socioeconomic status, and stage of disease. Prognostic factors should also be validated in several studies to ensure that there is a relationship between them and the outcome of interest.[9,12]

CRITICAL APPRAISAL OF AN ARTICLE

Box 1 lists key questions in the critical appraisal of an article on prognosis. The table is broken into three key sections, first looking at the methods, then the results, and finally the applicability of the study's results.[11]

RESEARCH METHODS
How Was the Study Designed?

Randomized-controlled trials (RCTs) are considered the "gold standard" for evaluating new drugs and medical or surgical procedures. However, it is uncommon to find RCTs assessing prognostic factors because of the ethical issues associated with assigning patients to potential risk factors,

---

Box 1
Evaluating an article on prognosis

I. Research methods
  i. How was the study designed?
  ii. Was the sample representative?
  iii. Is the sample group homogeneous with respect to prognostic factors?
  iv. Were measured outcomes unbiased and objective?
  v. Was follow-up complete?

II. Study results
  i. Does the article report the effect of prognostic/risk factors on outcome?
  ii. How precise are the reported estimates?

III. Applicability of study?
  i. Do the study patients match your own patients and was management similar?
  ii. Was the follow-up long enough?
  iii. Can the study results be used to help manage your patient?

for instance, randomizing patients to a healthy or unhealthy diet to examine effect on fracture healing in the hand.[13] Similarly, it would be unethical to randomize patients to smoking or nonsmoking if one were interested in determining the effect of smoking on skin viability following skin grafting.

Instead, surgical studies investigating prognostic factors are generally observational studies. The best such design is a cohort study; these may be either prospective or retrospective.[14] A prospective study identifies potential prognostic factors and follows study groups forward in time to determine whether any factors have a significant impact on outcomes. Unfortunately, these demand substantial planning in advance and require considerable time and resources to complete. An alternative is a retrospective cohort study or a retrospective case-control study, by far more common, which starts when an outcome has already been determined. In case-control studies, one starts with the outcome of interest and then looks backward to examine potential causal factors by comparing those who have the outcome (cases) with those who do not (controls). The major problem with retrospective studies is that the quality of the data is based mainly on patient records, which may not be sufficiently accurate. Retrospective studies are also prone to recall bias, which decreases the validity of their results.[11]

Was the Sample Representative?

The sample used in a study must match the target population. Any differences may introduce biases that may affect the incidence of adverse outcomes. Do the authors explicitly state what their population of interest is, and what their inclusion and exclusion criteria are? Do they describe the filters used to select candidates for the study? For instance, data on young patients in tertiary care, or major academic centers, may not be representative of a study examining the prognosis of young patients in the community, as tertiary care centers tend to accept patients with more complex conditions than those in peripheral community hospitals. Similarly, a study involving only patients treated at private clinics would not be representative of the general population, as these patients may have a different set of prognostic factors, in this case, socioeconomic status. A good article will give a clear description of how patients entered the study and the criteria used should be carefully spelled out, preferably at the outset, not buried within the body.

Is the Sample Group Homogeneous with Respect to Prognostic Factors?

The next step is to examine whether patients within the study are homogeneous with respect to prognostic risk. This is the ideal situation, as it decreases the potential for confounding factors. Are patients receiving the treatment for the same purpose (ie, the same preoperative diagnosis)? If not, it would be more precise to stratify the subjects into similar subgroups. This might provide more useful information for your specific patients, were he or she to fall into one of these categories allowing for a more precise estimate of risk. However, such specific studies may be difficult to find. In the case of clavicle fractures, it would be inappropriate to analyze data on very young children and elderly patients as a single cohort because, although the treatment may be the same, these two groups each carry their own set of characteristics that may affect their outcome.

Some prognostic studies that report on surgical outcomes will group the results of a few different techniques and report them as a single cohort. Although the injury being corrected is the same, with different surgeons using varying techniques or with different levels of skill, it becomes difficult to extract the prognostic value of a common variable. Whenever possible, studies should aim to have one surgeon conduct all procedures to eliminate these differences and allow for more accurate interpretation of the impact of the prognostic factors.

Were Measured Outcomes Unbiased and Objective?

Measured outcomes may be either objective or subjective. Objective outcomes do not depend on observer interpretation such as reoperation for nonunion or death. These either happen or they do not. Subjective outcomes require interpretation by assessors or patients and may be prone to problems with reliability on repeated measures. These include patient satisfaction, pain, and function after operation. Because these outcomes do offer important information on prognosis, authors should try to incorporate previously validated checklists and forms to measure them reliably. For example, the Disabilities of the Arm, Shoulder, and Hand (DASH) outcome measure is a self-report questionnaire that measures symptoms and disability in disorders of the upper limb. While subjective, it has been shown to be a reliable and valid test that clinicians can use to effectively assess upper extremity joints.[15] Similarly, the Michigan Hand Outcomes Questionnaire (MHQ), an instrument used in evaluation of outcomes following hand surgery, has undergone psychometric testing to prove its construct validity and reliability.[16]

Was Follow-Up Complete?

As Bhandari and colleagues[9] have explained, it is important to compare the proportion of patients lost to follow-up with those having had an adverse outcome. Without information on outcomes of patients lost, you cannot determine whether a surgery was successful, which will affect the estimate of true survival rate. One rule of thumb often used by clinicians, known as the "5 and 20" rule, states that a loss of more than 20% of patients significantly threatens the validity of a study's results, while a loss of less than 5% of patients produces a minimal or negligible effect on the results. This rule is merely a guide. The cases lost to follow-up should be considered as worst-case scenario results to determine if they could impact the studies' overall results.[11,17]

To illustrate numerically, consider a sample of 75 patients undergoing endoscopic carpal tunnel release procedures of whom 15 are lost to follow-up. Of the remaining patients, three required revision surgery. Omitting the lost patients from the analysis gives a reported failure rate of 5%. Because you are unsure of the outcome of those lost to follow-up, you cannot exclude the possibility that the failure to return resulted because surgery did not provide adequate pain relief. Were this the case, the overall failure rate would be greater than 5%, and possibly as great as 24% if all 15 were considered failures. At the other end, if the 15 lost patients were satisfied with their pain relief and felt no need to follow up (ie, did not have an adverse event), then the failure rate would be reduced to 4%. Given the multiple reasons for loss of patients, the true estimate of failure lies somewhere in between these two extremes. For these reasons, Randolph and colleagues[18] point out that loss of patients in follow-up is a potential source of bias.

As you can see, adding these results to the analysis significantly alters the treatment effect. Of course, if including lost patients as failures does not impact the magnitude of the treatment effect, then it is safe to say the inference made in the study is secure.[11]

Applying Study Design Criteria to Prognostic Studies on Distal Radius Fractures

When authors fail to provide information needed to adequately apply and assess some of the criteria in **Box 1**, a reader must judge whether they considered a particular point and failed to mention it, or whether they did not address it, which may compromise the validity of the study.[19]

In the first article identified in our search, Chung and colleagues[7] used a prospective cohort design to identify predictors of outcomes after surgical treatment of distal radius fractures. Patients were identified at the time of injury with inclusion and exclusion criteria explicitly stated. Inclusion criteria were kept broad and explanations for exclusion were provided.

Attempts were made to keep the sample homogeneous as well. Surgical techniques and postoperative management were similar for each patient, although it was not clear whether the same surgeon had operated on all patients. All procedures were performed at the University of Michigan Medical Center. Defined radiological criteria were used for qualification for surgical fixation.

Primary outcomes were measured with the Michigan Hand Questionnaire (MHQ), which although subjective and self-reported, is a validated hand-specific tool. The MHQ generates a score based on function, pain, aesthetics, and patient satisfaction. Secondary outcome measures were based on AP and lateral radiographs of the wrist, and categorization of fracture by the Orthopaedic Trauma Association classification. Patients were evaluated at 3 months, 6 months, and 1 year by the treating hand surgeon, as well as by a physician's assistant, who looked for the presence of complications. From a total of 93 patients originally enrolled in the study, data were available for 66 at 3 months and 49 at 1 year. The mean age of the patients was 49 ± 17 years. Although complete follow-up data were not available for all patients, the researchers did compare baseline characteristics between those lost and those followed and found no statistically or clinically significant differences between the groups.

This study has high validity, and is a prospective cohort design. The sample is representative of adult patients with an isolated injury who present at a tertiary care center after distal radius fracture, since few filters were used. Many prognostic factors were identified and the population was split into subgroups, which were analyzed through multiple regression analysis.

In the second article, Rozental and Blazar[8] followed 49 patients with distal radius fractures who were treated with volar locking plates between 2002 and 2004. It was not stated who performed the operations or at which centers. Patients were retrospectively identified through a chart review and followed forward in time, measuring both functional outcome and radiographic outcomes of the operative procedure. Information was collected on the patients' age, mechanism of injury, and AO classification of their fracture.

Of the original subset of 49 patients, 8 patients were excluded either because they were followed for less than 1 year or had also been treated with dorsal plating or external fixation. The remaining 41 were followed for a minimum of 1 year, with average follow-up duration being 17 months. A brief description of the operative procedure for application of the volar plate was provided. The outcome measures of interest included functional range of motion measured with a goniometer, and radiographic measurement of radial inclination, radial length, and volar tilt. These outcomes were measured at the latest follow-up date by one of the two authors, who was, as a result, not blinded. However, outcome results involved the use of measurement tools, thus decreasing potential observer bias.

For this study, a representative sample was identified, follow-up was sufficient, and outcome measures were objective. However authors failed to examine the influence of prognostic factors on outcome and did not control for the surgeons' choice of volar plate design. Therefore, there are some concerns with this article's validity.

STUDY RESULTS
Does the Article Report the Effect of Prognostic/Risk Factors on Outcome?

Once a study has been judged to provide valid information regarding its design, the reader may then extract information regarding the effect of prognostic factors on survival rates and procedural outcomes. Surgical studies monitoring outcomes should report on the number of failures or adverse events over a period of time, which can be used to create Kaplan-Meier curves. These survival curves provide a nonparametric estimate of the probability of success of the surgery over a certain number of years.[18] It is also important that an article report both positive and negative outcomes together with their associated circumstances. For instance, in an article describing outcomes after total ankle arthroplasty by Spirt and colleagues,[20] only failures were reported, with no information provided to describe the successful outcomes. This article would be useful if a patient had many factors in common with the failure group but would provide little useful information for a patient whose prognosis looks promising.[18]

How Precise Are the Reported Estimates?

Estimates are commonly described using confidence intervals (CI), which instead of being point estimates, are a range of values likely to include the parameter being examined. The narrower the CI, the more precise the estimate is. For a specified level of confidence there are only two ways to decrease the width: to increase the sample size or to reduce variation among the subjects. There are practical considerations that limit the sample size

while variation among the subjects can be reduced only by proper experimental design, a methodology that is not readily available in case-control or cohort studies. Typically, papers will mention relative risk or odds ratio, and it is common to provide 95% CI. This means that if the same study were performed 100 times then the true parameter of interest for the entire population would lie within the confidence interval produced by the sample in approximately 95% of the studies, or 19 times out of 20.

Applying to Our Studies

The article by Chung and colleagues[7] reported on a substantial number of prognostic factors, including baseline characteristics (age, gender, income, education, dominant hand fractured, workers compensation, AO fracture classification) and postoperative radiographic measures (volar-tilt angle, radial height, radial inclination, and total incongruity). They used a multiple regression analysis with the baseline and radiographic demographics as independent variables, and overall MHQ scores as the dependent variable. They performed separate analyses for 3 months and 1 year, but also used a model to combine the two to pull strength from multiple measurements over time, which accounts for potential within-patient correlation. They reported on 10 complications, ranging from skin irritation to hardware protrusion to subsequent carpal tunnel release, with an incidence of 12.6% over the 1-year period. However, the complications were not analyzed to identify risk factors for complication, as the main outcome was MHQ score. In their final analysis, only age and income significantly altered outcomes after 1 year, with each year increase in age associated with a 0.29 decrease in MHQ score (95% CI −0.53 to 0.04). A significant improvement was seen in outcomes between 3 months and 1 year ($P < .01$) after adjusting for fracture type and age. Finally, all other prognostic factors were not found to be significant at the 1-year follow-up, including fracture severity, hand dominance, or postoperative radiographic measures.

In the article by Rozental and Blazar,[8] all patients in the study had satisfactory reduction of their fracture postoperatively and at their latest follow-up, defined as less than 10 degrees of dorsal tilt, less than 2 mm of radial shortening, and less than 1 mm of articular incongruity. They also all achieved a minimum range of motion arc of 60 degrees for flexion/extension and 144 degrees for supination/pronation. Seven percent of patients had hardware complications requiring re-operation. In this study, the authors failed to address the outcome results for specific subgroups based on prognostic factors, preventing the reader from being able to apply these results accurately to his or her patient. The results thus estimate the success rates of fracture repair for a heterogeneous group of patients, which limits the study's overall applicability.[9]

APPLICABILITY OF STUDY
Do the Study Patients Match Your Own Patients and Was Management Similar?

A study must provide a sufficient description of the subjects before a surgeon can decide that it is applicable to his or her own patient. It should address which characteristics were monitored and if these variables were incorporated as a subanalysis when reporting results.

Furthermore, a study should use similar management to your own to provide consistent data that can then be extrapolated and applied to your patient. Consider the treatment of anterior shoulder dislocations; if a study aims to compare two reduction techniques for the highest first-attempt reduction rate, if no mention is made of the method of analgesia or sedation for each dislocation, how can a reader gauge the ease of reduction?[21] In the reader's own practice, he or she is left guessing. The management cannot be deemed similar from case to case, leaving the results with limited applicability.

Was the Follow-Up Long Enough?

It is difficult to define a single length of time that would constitute an adequate follow-up, as this time is a function of the type of procedure investigated. While shorter duration is appropriate for studies investigating outcomes such as time to fracture union or surgical site infections in plastic surgery procedures,[22] longer periods are required when investigating the survival of an implant, such as a hip prosthesis. Measuring functional outcomes postoperatively would also warrant a longer follow-up period.

A practical consideration is that that surgery is a rapidly evolving field and what is considered the standard of care today, may be outdated in 15 years. Long-term follow-up data for a procedure that is no longer used, therefore becomes less relevant. A balance must be attained between reporting on long-term outcomes and providing information that is applicable to current surgical techniques.

Can the Study Results Be Used to Help Manage Your Patient?

When a study reveals certain prognostic factors to significantly influence the outcome of a proposed treatment, the surgeon then has a solid basis on which to make a decision of choice of treatment. For example, intra-medullary (IM) nailing is considered the standard of care for femoral shaft fractures. However, in patients involved in traumatic accidents with multiple other injuries, including increased intracranial pressure (ICP), external fixation may be used as a bridging technique until the patient is stable enough for nailing. So while IM nailing is generally the gold standard, the risk factor of increased ICP, associated with a poor outcome in IM nailing,[23] may alter the physician's treatment choice.

Even when the results of a study do not definitively help with selection of appropriate therapy, they may still be useful in providing a starting point for consulting with colleagues or in counseling a patient.[11] Perhaps surgery is not warranted because of patient risk factors, or the natural history of the disease is so benign that surgery is unnecessary. Having evidence to support your options or choices may ease your patient's concerns. Prognostic study outcomes can also be helpful for the surgeon with his or her own concerns about success rates and prognosis of the treatment. Conclusions drawn from study results may lead to a positive conversation if the prognosis is good, or to end-of-life care discussions if the prognosis is grim.

RESOLUTION OF THE SCENARIO

Our review of the study by Chung and colleagues[7] indicates that it has fairly high validity. It is a prospective cohort design with a sample that is representative of adult patients with an isolated injury who present at a tertiary care center after distal radius fracture. As few filters were used, our patient's characteristics do not exclude him from the population of subjects from whom the sample was taken and were enrolled in the study. Many prognostic factors were identified and the population was split into subgroups, which were analyzed through multiple regression, enabling us to apply more specific data to our patient. Patients were followed for a year, allowing the investigators to report on short-term complications.

Referring back to our patient's questions, with these results we can confidently inform him that, although his fracture was severe and in his dominant hand, he should experience no worse an outcome than if it were a simpler fracture occurring in his nondominant hand. In addressing his concerns about age, we can inform him only that increasing age is associated with a poorer functional outcome, as demonstrated with lower MHQ scores, although the article did not indicate how to convert the raw MHQ scores into an actual level of function. However, the study still would allow us to give our patient some idea of what he should expect after his surgery.

The study by Rozental and Blazar[8] fails to specify how prognostic factors affect the functional outcome of patients undergoing volar plating. The authors fail to control the selection of the design of the volar plate, as this was surgeon's preference. Also, the patients were identified through a retrospective chart review, which decreases the validity of the study design. Therefore, for these reasons the results are not as applicable as the results from the first article.

The following day in your office, you explain your findings to the patient, who is relieved that he will be able to return to his active, independent lifestyle after the operation.

SUMMARY

We have presented an approach to appraising a prognostic study using the example of prognosis following surgical reduction of a distal radius fracture. We have identified a set of questions a reader should keep in mind when evaluating the clinical importance of a research finding with particular attention to applicability of results to his or her own patients. With time and continued practice, such critical appraisal of articles will become automatic, providing physicians with the ability to select relevant articles from the vast resources of published information and the tools to make informed, evidence-based clinical decisions.

REFERENCES

1. Guyatt G. Evidence-based medicine: past, present and future. McMaster Univ Med J 2003;1:27–32.
2. Evidence-Based Medicine Working Group. Evidence-based medicine: a new approach to teaching the practice of medicine. JAMA 1992;268:2420–5.
3. Gehrmann SV, Windolf J, Kaufmann RA. Distal radius fracture management in elderly patients: a literature review. J Hand Surg [Am] 2008;33A:421–9.
4. Singer BR, McLauchlan GJ, Robinson CM, et al. Epidemiology of fractures in 15,000 adults: the influence of age and gender. J Bone Joint Surg Br 1998;80B(2):243–8.
5. Ruch DS, Papdonikolakis A. Volar versus dorsal plating in the management of intra-articular distal radius fractures. J Hand Surg 2006;31(1):9–16.
6. Osada D, Viegas SF, Shah MA, et al. Comparison of different distal radius dorsal and volar fracture fixation plates: a biomechanical study. J Hand Surg 2003;28(1):94–104.
7. Chung KC, Kotsis SV, Kim M. Predictors of functional outcomes after surgical treatment of distal radius fractures. J Hand Surg [Am] 2007;32A(1):76–82.
8. Rozental TD, Blazar PE. Functional outcome and complications after volar plating for dorsally displaced, unstable fractures of the distal radius. J Hand Surg 2006;31A(3):359–64.
9. Bhandari M, Guyatt GH, Swiontkowski MF. User's guide to the orthopaedic literature: how to use an article about prognosis. J Bone Joint Surg Am 2001;83-A(10):1555–64.
10. Radwin RG, Sesto ME, Zachary SV. Functional tests to quantify recovery following carpal tunnel release. J Bone Joint Surg Am 2004;86-A(12):2614–20.
11. Guyatt G, Rennie D. Users' guide to the medical literature: essentials of evidence-based clinical practice. Chicago: American Medical Association Press; 2001.
12. Bhandari M, Devereaux PJ, Montori V, et al. Users' guide to the surgical literature: how to use a systematic literature review and meta-analysis. Can J Surg 2004;47(1):60–7.
13. LaStayo PC, Winters KM, Hardy M. Fracture healing: bone healing, fracture management, and current concepts related to the hand. J Hand Ther 2003;16(2):81–94.
14. Thoma A, Farrokhyar F, Bhandari M, et al. Users' guide to the surgical literature: how to assess a randomized controlled trial in surgery. Can J Surg 2004;47(3):200–8.
15. Beaton DE, Katz JN, Fossel AH, et al. Measuring the whole or the parts? Validity, reliability, and responsiveness of the disabilities of the arm, shoulder and hand outcome measure in different regions of the upper extremity. J Hand Ther 2001;14(2):128–46.
16. Chung KC, Pillsbury MS, Walters MR, et al. Reliability and validity testing of the Michigan hand outcomes questionnaire. J Hand Surg 1998;23(4):575–87.
17. Haynes RB, Strauss SE. Evidence-based medicine: how to practice and teach EBM. Edinburgh, New York: Elsevier/Churchill Livingstone; 2005.
18. Randolph A, Bucher H, Richardson S, et al. In: Guyatt G, Rennie D, editors. Users' guide to the medical literature: essentials of evidence-based clinical practice. Chicago: American Medical Association Press; 2001.
19. Hoppe DJ, Degen RM, Bhandari M. User's guide to a prognostic study on an orthopaedic implant. J Long Term Eff Med Implants 2007;17(2):135–44.
20. Spirt AA, Assal M, Hansent ST Jr. Complications and failure after total ankle arthroplasty. J Bone Joint Surg Am 2004;86-A(6):1172–8.
21. Beattie TF, Steedman J, McGowan A, et al. A comparison of the Milch and Kocher techniques for

acute anterior dislocation of the shoulder. Injury 1986;17:349–52.

22. Drapeau CM, D'Aniello C, Brafa A, et al. Surgical site infections in plastic surgery: an Italian multicenter study. J Surg Res 2007;143(2):393–7.

23. Scalea TM, Boswell SA, Scott JD, et al. External fixation as a bridge to intramedullary nailing for patients with multiple injuries and with femur fractures: damage control orthopedics. J Trauma: Injury, Infection and Critical Care 2000;48(4):613–23.

Evaluating Equivalency of Treatment Effectiveness: The Example of Arthroscopic and Mini-Open Rotator Cuff Repairs

Helen Razmjou, MSc, PT, PhD(C)[a,b,*]

KEYWORDS

• Rotator cuff repair • Mini-open • Arthroscopy

The evidence-based practice (EBP) involves integrating expertise and judgment with the best available external evidence and patient values into the process of care.[1] There are many challenges clinicians face to practice or teach evidence-based medicine. A simple example is choosing the best surgical treatment in the absence of sufficient evidence and in the fast evolving world of technology where new instruments and techniques are being introduced to orthopaedic surgeons on a regular basis.

With the increasing interest in using less invasive surgeries, arthroscopic rotator cuff repairs have become fairly popular. All-arthroscopic surgery has improved the ability of the orthopaedic surgeons to visualize, mobilize, and secure the torn tendons. There are a number of advantages to using arthroscopic rotator cuff repairs, including: improved cosmesis; less disturbance of the deltoid musculature; improved infection rates; the possibility of detecting associated glenohumeral or labral pathologies; less pain and stiffness; shortened hospital stay; and accelerated rehabilitation. The arguments against arthroscopic repairs include: higher costs related to more expensive equipments; more difficulty achieving technical skills; and the potential for less secured repairs.[2–9]

The limited studies that have compared all-arthroscopic surgery with mini-open repairs do not provide definitive conclusions because of the retrospective nature of the studies, small or unequal sample sizes, lack of clear hypothesis or a priori quantitative boundary for what would constitute "equivalence" or "superiority," and absence of cogent analytic methods.[10] This article uses the principle of critical appraisal within an EBP framework to evaluate the literature in this area.

PRESENT STATE OF KNOWLEDGE

Currently, there are no randomized controlled trials (RCT) or prospective cohort studies comparing the mini-open to all-arthroscopic techniques in patients with full-thickness rotator cuff tears. There are a number of retrospective cohort studies that have compared the results of the two techniques.[2–9]

A systematic review of the literature[11] that has compared clinical outcomes of mini-open with all-arthroscopic techniques of rotator cuff repair shows that both arthroscopic and mini-open rotator cuff repairs result in significant clinical

a Holland Orthopaedic and Arthritic Centre, Sunnybrook Health Sciences Centre, 43 Wellesley Street East, Toronto, Ontario M1Y 1H1, Canada
b Women's College Research Institute, 790 Bay Street, Toronto, Ontario M5G 1N8, Canada
* Holland Orthopaedic and Arthritic Centre, Sunnybrook Health Sciences Centre, 43 Wellesley Street East, Toronto, Ontario M1Y 1H1, Canada.
E-mail address: helen.razmjou@sunnybrook.ca

Hand Clin 25 (2009) 67–70
doi:10.1016/j.hcl.2008.10.002
0749-0712/08/$ – see front matter © 2009 Elsevier Inc. All rights reserved.

improvement, with relatively low complication rates. Although a slightly increased rate of complications was reported with the mini-open repair, the authors could not identify a significant difference between the two techniques.[11]

Although a systematic review is considered the highest level of evidence, when studies fail to detect differences between the groups, the authors' concern about power and other quality issues should be heightened. In these studies, conclusions that two methods were equivalent in outcome were often drawn based on *P* values and a lack of statistical significance. However, the majority of the previous studies: did not differentiate between "equivalence" and "superiority;" failed to set a quantitative boundary for the magnitude of effect size; did not use an adequate sample to detect a meaningful clinically important difference between groups; and lacked rigorous statistical analysis to support the equivalence claim. Failure to detect a difference between outcomes of two surgical treatments does not necessarily imply equivalence and such an approach is likely to lead to the wrong conclusions, such as underestimating the effect of one procedure over the other.[10,12,13]

A detailed discussion of the definition and implications of "equivalence studies" is beyond the scope of this paper. However, before examining the available literature on all-arthroscopic and mini-open repairs of the rotator cuff, a summary of methodological criteria that need to be considered when assessing accuracy of "no difference" or "equivalence" claims made in clinical trials is provided.[10]

- First, and most importantly, it is expected that the investigators note their goal of detecting superiority or equivalence in the statement of their research aim as a priori hypothesis. It is not sufficient to simply state: "our aim is to compare treatment A with treatment B." The purpose of an equivalence trial is to establish identical effects of the therapies being compared. A superiority trial aims to demonstrate the superiority of the new surgery compared with a more established surgery. The choice of research aim affects hypothesis and sample size calculation. The statistical tests for superiority are aimed at rejecting a null hypothesis of "no difference" whereas a test of equivalency is intended to reject the "alternative" hypothesis.
- Secondly, sample size should be justified based on the hypothesis. The sample size justification in orthopedics is usually based on subjective outcomes. These outcomes should

have established reliability and validity to be able to detect small and clinically important differences between groups. Unfortunately, subjective disability questionnaires that document functional and emotional difficulty related to orthopedic related problems have large standard deviations that demand large number of patients, especially two years postoperatively, a desired end point for most surgical journals. In superiority trials, sample size is based on the minimal clinically important difference or the effect size denoted by δ. The variance of the effect variable is usually obtained from a pilot study or previous literature. Although it is desirable to have zero type I (false positive) and type II (false negative) errors, because of limited resources, small risks of error is acceptable ($\alpha = 5\%$ for type I error) and ($\beta = 10–20\%$ for type II error). The complimentary probability for β is $(1-\beta)$, which indicates the power of the trial because it states the probability of finding δ if the difference truly exists. When intending to prove that two treatments are no different, the conventional sample size formula used for superiority trials is not appropriate due to interchanging the hypothesis and error types.[13]

For establishing complete equivalent effects, an effect size (δ) value of zero is assumed and because this is not possible, the difference in effects between two surgeries should lie within a specified small interval chosen by investigators. Because δ has to be very small, the sample size of the equivalence studies is much larger than superiority trials, which clinicians and researchers should bear in mind. Most often, the sample sizes of equivalence trials are four times more than a corresponding superiority trial.[13]

- *Setting up quantitative boundaries* for effect size is as important as having an appropriate sample size. The *P* values should not be the only criterion for claiming significant differences between groups. With large sample sizes, *P* values become significant without having any clinical implications. Similarly, small samples often seen in surgical trials fail to detect true differences between two surgical procedures. Unfortunately, some investigators declare equivalence after a failed test for superiority. The claim of equivalence may well be misleading if an observed important distinction is not confirmed just because the sample size is too small. Conclusions should be drawn on the basis of an appropriate confidence interval using the previously specified criteria of equivalence.[10,12–14]

Table 1
Summary of comparative studies on arthroscopic and mini-open repair of rotator cuffs

Authors	Design	Subjects	Mean FU	Outcome Measures / Effect Size	Hypothesis	Sample Size	Quantitative Boundaries	Analysis
Kim et al, 2003	Retrospective	42/34	39 M	ASES: 0.17 UCLA: 0.38	Not stated	Not justified	Not stated	P values
Severud et al, 2003	Retrospective	35/29	45 M	ASES[a] UCLA[a]	Not stated	Not justified	Not stated	P values
Ide et al, 2005	Retrospective	50/50	49 M	UCLA[a] JOA[a]	Not stated	Not justified	Not stated	P values
Warner et al, 2005	Retrospective	9/12	27 M	SST[a] Stiffness[a]	Equivalence Superiority	Not justified	Not stated	P values
Sauerbrey et al, 2005	Retrospective	28/26	26 M	ASES[a]	Not stated	Not justified	Not stated	P values
Youm et al, 2005	Retrospective	42/42	24 M	ASES: 0.07 UCLA: 0.27	Not stated	Not justified	Not stated	P values
Verma et al, 2006	Retrospective	38/33	24 M	ASES: 0.05 SST: 0.07 L'Insalata: 017	Equivalence	Based on superiority	Not stated	P values
Kang et al, 2007	Retrospective	65/63	6 M	SST: 0.44 DASH: 0.02 SF36 (8 domains) VAS (pain, function, quality of life)	Equivalence	Not justified	Not stated	P values

[a] Effect size (difference between groups divided by the standard deviation of the control [mini-open] group) could not be calculated due to lack of information on standard deviation.

Abbreviations: ASES, American Shoulder & Elbow Surgeons; DASH, disabilities of the arm, shoulder and hand; JOA, Japanese Orthopaedic Association; UCLA, University of California Los Angeles; VAS, visual analogue scale.

- Rigorous statistical testing is the other important attribute of claiming no difference in outcomes between two surgical treatments. The conclusions should examine whether the differences observed between groups or patients are compared with a specific confidence interval boundary rather than a significant *P* value that changes with sample size.

The information on the treatment of rotator cuff repairs is limited at this point, mostly because of a lack of randomized controlled trials and prospective cohort studies. The only systematic review of the literature in this area[11] was not able to provide a quantitative systematic review and meta-analysis because of shortcomings of previous studies and lack of RCT studies. The limited retrospective or matched case studies report no difference between two surgeries.[2–9] **Table 1** presents a summary of the literature related to arthroscopic and mini-open studies with respect to methodological criteria required for equivalence studies. Out of eight original comparative studies, only three studies stated their hypothesis clearly.[3,7,8] The sample sizes for each surgical arm varied from nine to fifty subjects,[2,8] which raises questions about the power of the study in detecting any important difference regardless of the outcome measure used. Some of these studies did not even provide a standard deviation for readers to calculate the magnitude of the effect size.[2,5,6,8] Only one retrospective study noted a priori hypothesis, justified their sample size based on minimal clinically important change of a joint specific questionnaire, provided the American Shoulder and Elbow Surgeons (ASES) score, and provided enough information for readers to examine the effect size between treatments.[7] In this study, the hypothesis was that "no difference would be seen in clinical outcomes of two surgeries." However, the sample size was based on conventional power calculation used for superiority trials (aiming to detect 7% difference in ASES scores), which significantly underestimates the number of subjects.

In summary, lack of evidence on superiority of arthroscopy over mini-open or vice versa indicates a major need for improvement in the quality of published studies in this area. Surgeons should be aware that the equivalence option is an important concept for surgical trials as it is often the case that less invasive procedures need to show equivalent primary outcomes to be accepted. However, if the research question is truly one of equivalence, research design issues should be evaluated on this basis. Lack of superiority is not an indication of equivalence. Future research should focus on prospective, randomized clinical trials with pre-specified hypotheses, proper sample sizes, validated outcome measures, and confirmatory postoperative imaging studies.

REFERENCES

1. Sackett DL, Rosenberg WM, Gray JA, et al. Evidence based medicine: what it is and what it isn't. BMJ 1996;312(7023):71–2.
2. Ide J, Maeda S, Takagi K. A comparison of arthroscopic and open rotator cuff repair. Arthroscopy 2005;21(9):1090–8.
3. Kang L, Henn RF, Tashjian RZ, et al. Early outcome of arthroscopic rotator cuff repair: a matched comparison with mini-open rotator cuff repair. Arthroscopy 2007;23(6):573–82, 582.e1–2.
4. Kim SH, Ha KI, Park JH, et al. Arthroscopic versus mini-open salvage repair of the rotator cuff tear: outcome analysis at 2 to 6 years' follow-up. Arthroscopy 2003;19(7):746–54.
5. Sauerbrey AM, Getz CL, Piancastelli M, et al. Arthroscopic versus mini-open rotator cuff repair: a comparison of clinical outcome. Arthroscopy 2005; 21(12):1415–20.
6. Severud EL, Ruotolo C, Abbott DD, et al. All-arthroscopic versus mini-open rotator cuff repair: a long-term retrospective outcome comparison. Arthroscopy 2003;19(3):234–8.
7. Verma NN, Dunn W, Adler RS, et al. All-arthroscopic versus mini-open rotator cuff repair: a retrospective review with minimum 2-year follow-up. Arthroscopy 2006;22(6):587–94.
8. Warner JJ, Tetreault P, Lehtinen J, et al. Arthroscopic versus mini-open rotator cuff repair: a cohort comparison study. Arthroscopy 2005;21(3):328–32.
9. Youm T, Murray DH, Kubiak EN, et al. Arthroscopic versus mini-open rotator cuff repair: a comparison of clinical outcomes and patient satisfaction. J Shoulder Elbow Surg 2005;14(5):455–9.
10. Greene WL, Concato J, Feinstein AR. Claims of equivalence in medical research: are they supported by the evidence? Ann Intern Med 2000;132(9):715–22.
11. Nho SJ, Shindle MK, Sherman SL, et al. Systematic review of arthroscopic rotator cuff repair and mini-open rotator cuff repair. J Bone Joint Surg Am 2007;89(Suppl. 3):127–36.
12. Gomberg-Maitland M, Frison L, Halperin JL. Active-control clinical trials to establish equivalence or non-inferiority: methodological and statistical concepts linked to quality. Am Heart J 2003;146(3):398–403.
13. Christensen E. Methodology of superiority vs. equivalence trials and non-inferiority trials. J Hepatol 2007;46(5):947–54.
14. Tinmouth JM, Steele LS, Tomlinson G, et al. Are claims of equivalency in digestive diseases trials supported by the evidence? Gastroenterology 2004;126(7):1700–10.

Measuring Quality in Health Care and Its Implications for Pay-For-Performance Initiatives

Kevin C. Chung, MD, MS*, Melissa J. Shauver, MPH

KEYWORDS

- Quality • Health care • Pay-for-performance
- Hand surgery • Outcomes

Health care is a decisive issue in the 2008 United States presidential election. Over the past months, the candidates' visions for future health care policies have been discussed, debated, and dissected. In a December 2007 poll by the Kaiser Family Foundation, health care ranked second on a list of voters' most important issues.[1] It is so important that 21% of Americans named health care as the single most important issue in their choice for president in this election.[1] In contrast, in 2004, health care ranked only fourth among decisive issues, with only 14% of those polled considering it the most important.[2] The issue of health care has remained a major concern because restrictions and lack of access to affordable care have eroded the standard of living expected by many Americans.

Any discussion of health care is likely to touch on a trio of topics: cost, access, and quality. These topics weigh on the minds of health care consumers. A September 2007 CBS News poll found that 66% of registered voters reported that they were unsatisfied with the quality of health care in the United States.[3] Another recent poll by the Kaiser Family Foundation found that 80% of respondents were worried about the worsening of the quality of the health care services they receive.[4] Furthermore, 81% of Americans reported that they were dissatisfied with the cost of health care in the United States, up from 62% in 2004 (**Fig. 1**).[2,3]

There is much about which to be dissatisfied. United States health care spending is among the highest in the world, averaging $7026 per person, or $2.1 trillion in 2006, and is growing at a rate of over 6.7% per year.[5–7] Despite continually increasing expenditures, the United States has not enjoyed the quality that should be accompanied by this enormous investment (**Fig. 2**).[6] The stakes are high for various special interests groups to protect their "turfs" in this battle for health care allocations. These interest groups, which include the government, insurance companies, health maintenance organizations, consumer groups (eg, the American Association of Retired Persons), employees of corporations, and ordinary consumers, have competing interests that conflict with hospitals and physician organizations in their efforts to extract as much as possible from a fixed pie of health care expenditure.

The current system of United States medical care is based on the free-market economic model

This article is supported in part by a grant from the National Institute of Arthritis and Musculoskeletal and Skin Diseases (R01 AR047328) and a Midcareer Investigator Award in Patient-Oriented Research (K24 AR053120) (to K.C. Chung).

Section of Plastic Surgery, Department of Surgery, The University of Michigan Health System, 2130 Taubman Center, SPC 5340, 1500 East Medical Center Drive, Ann Arbor, MI, 48109–5340, USA

* Corresponding author.

E-mail address: kecchung@umich.edu (K.C. Chung).

Hand Clin 25 (2009) 71–81
doi:10.1016/j.hcl.2008.09.001

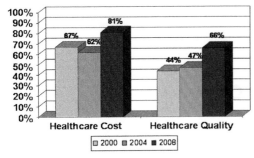

Fig. 1. Percent of Americans dissatisfied with United States health care costs and United States health care quality. (*Data from* Kaiser health tracking poll: election 2008. Menlo Park (CA): The Henry J. Kaiser Family Foundation; 2007; and Health care and the Democratic presidential campaign: CBS News; September 17, 2007; and Kaiser Family Foundation poll. Storrs (CT): Roper Center for Public Opinion Research; 2007.)

in which supply and demand create a mutually beneficial market for both buyers and sellers. Noted Princeton University health economist Uwe Reinhardt supports this free-market model. He believes that competition in medicine is healthy and has the potential to give consumers the ability to choose among various providers for the highest quality of care.[8] He also realizes, however, that medicine is a unique field, influenced by government regulation, consumer norms, and market prices.[8] In addition to not holding price in check, the existing United States provider reimbursement system does not pay much attention to quality, but

bases payment instead on volume and intensity of services provided.[9,10] As the United States moves toward a single-payor system like those that have been adopted by many industrialized nations, quality metrics will be instituted to improve efficiency of service delivery by focusing on preventive care measures and minimizing costly complications.[11]

EVOLUTION OF THE UNITED STATES HEALTH CARE SYSTEM

Before the 1970s, private and public payors reimbursed physicians and hospitals customary fees for their services. Charges were submitted to the insurance carriers, who typically paid the full amount. As the cost of health care continued to rise, however, Medicare and private insurers adopted the diagnostic-related groups, which introduced the concept of fixed case-rate payment. Rather than paying hospitals for each test and procedure individually, specific payment rates were given to hospitals based on diagnosis.[10] The diagnostic-related groups introduced the concept of capitation, which shifted the financial burden to the hospitals. The aim of the diagnostic-related group system is to encourage hospitals to discharge patients earlier and to curb the ordering of expensive, often optional, tests. Because hospitals are paid a set amount, if they can practice medicine more cost-effectively, they will retain more of their reimbursement. The diagnostic-related group model had a great effect in reducing the length-of-stay in hospitals. For example, in

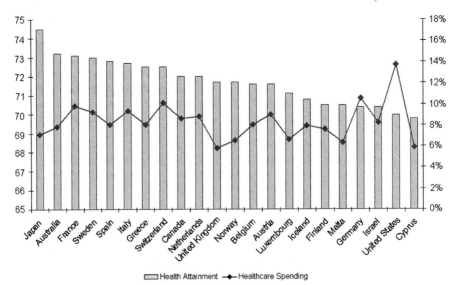

Fig. 2. Health attainment (disability-adjusted life expectancy) and health care spending (percent of GDP). (*Data from* The world health report 2000. Health systems: improving performance. Available at: http://www.who.int/whr/2000/en/whr00_en.pdf. Accessed March 3, 2008.)

the past, patients who underwent elective surgical procedures may have been admitted to the hospital for a few days before preoperative evaluations. With pressure placed on hospitals to discharge patients earlier, minimally invasive procedures, such as laparoscopic operations, have become much more popular. Additionally, preoperative tests and evaluations are now performed in an outpatient setting. Many surgical procedures have shifted from inpatient to outpatient facilities as a consequence.

The resource-based relative value scale introduced in the late 1980s was another attempt to decrease health care costs by limiting physician payment through a metric of intensity of their services.[12] Although the resource-based relative value scale system aimed to curb physician payment, it could induce an increased use of services by physicians to make up for the decrease in payments. Finally, the proliferation of health maintenance organizations temporarily decreased health care expenditures by decreasing health care coverage and capitating physician payments. This was done by shifting the financial responsibilities onto the physicians, whereas the executives of certain health maintenance organizations have reaped large profits at the expense of the American people.[13] The imposition of the "take it or leave it" positions by the health maintenance organizations in setting their fee schedule hampered physicians' ability to receive fair payments for their services because of antitrust limitations on physicians' contract negotiations.[14] It is quite apparent that these failed initiatives to curb health care costs have made physicians and the general public view this quality movement with great skepticism. The true intentions of this initiative have been called into question by some, pinning it as yet another intrusion into physician autonomy and a veiled attempted in cutting physician income.

The Institute of Medicine (IOM), a branch of the National Academy of Sciences, provides scientifically informed, nonbiased analysis and advice to policy makers, medical professionals, and the general public.[15] The IOM presented two important publications to highlight the quality problems in American medicine. The first of these publications is "To Err is Human," in which the IOM estimated that as many as 98,000 deaths per year in the United States are caused by medical error.[16] In subsequent discussions, the IOM gave recommendations regarding improving the American health care system through the paper "Crossing the Quality Chasm: A New Health System for the 21st century."[17] In this paper, the IOM emphasizes that the gap between the current state of American health care and what is needed has widened. This chasm is caused by changing health care needs; new and increased use of technology; and the growth in the elderly population, who often have chronic conditions.[17] To begin remedying this situation, the IOM recommended the following: (1) applying evidence to health care delivery, (2) using information technology more appropriately, (3) better training for health care workforce, and (4) aligning payment with quality improvement.[17] Clearly, there is much room for improvement in the quality of American health care.

DEFINITION OF HEALTH CARE QUALITY

Before any discussion of health care quality can begin, one must define what, exactly, is quality. Although the definition has evolved over the years, the IOM's definition is the most widely used.[18] Published in 1990, the IOM's definition states that quality is "the degree to which health services for individuals and populations increase the likelihood of desired health outcomes and are consistent with current professional knowledge."[17] This straightforward definition masks the difficulty of actually measuring health care quality.

The measurement of health care quality is fraught with potholes and paradoxes. First, there are numerous stakeholders (providers, patients, health care organizations, insurers, purchasers of health care) each with their own interests to protect, often conflicting with other stakeholders. Second, it is virtually impossible to create a completely error-free measure that is applicable to every situation.[19] Finally, the demands placed on quality measures are often unrealistic. Donabedian,[20] a pioneer in the field of health care quality measurement, observed that those who are not familiar with quality assessment "demand measures that are easy, precise, and complete – as if a sack of potatoes being weighed."

MEASUREMENT OF HEALTH CARE QUALITY

Quality can be assessed in one of three domains: (1) structure, (2) process, and (3) outcome. Structural assessments are based on the attributes of the setting in which the care is received. These attributes may be of the physician (eg, specialty or years in practice); the hospital (staffing characteristics, facilities); or the health care system as a whole (financial resources, staff organization).[20] Process denotes components of the encounter between patient and health care provider (ie, what actions were taken by both patient and provider).[20] For example, process measures may include whether compression stockings are placed for long operations or whether a preoperative time-out is instituted to avoid wrong-site surgery. Outcome assessments are, quite simply, the status of the patient following care.[20] Outcomes may include health-related quality of life or morbidity and mortality rates.

Outcome assessment was one of the first measures of health care quality. In 1916, Ernest Amory Codman, the father of the modern outcomes movement, had suggested methods to monitor what he termed "end results" of care.[21] For certain procedures or conditions, however, outcomes measures can be quite elusive. Outcomes after carpal tunnel release, for example, cannot be measured accurately with physical tests, such as grip strength or range of motion. Assessment of these outcomes must be based on patient-rated instruments by assessing patients' perception of their symptom and functional improvement. For other procedures, such as silicone arthroplasty, certain complications (eg, joint loosening) may take many years to develop, making it difficult for surgeons and therapists to determine this procedure's effectiveness unless the patients are followed for many years after surgery.

These difficulties have led health analysts to turn toward structure and process measures as a proxy of quality of care. Many structure and process measures can be assessed relatively easily and precisely. Information on institution procedure volume or the practice of administrating preoperative antibiotics is readily available or can be abstracted from patient charts with little difficulty. Because of their straightforward nature, these are generally thought to be adequate quality measures;[19] however, there are drawbacks. Outcomes do not always suffer, despite poor performance on structure and process measures. Most patients do not develop wound infections, even for those who do not receive prophylactic antibiotics. Just because these patients do not experience poor outcomes, because of luck alone, ought not to indicate that they receive high-quality care. One must be careful not to confuse a lack of negative outcomes with good quality of care.

MEASURING SURGICAL QUALITY

Quality can be assessed both explicitly and implicitly. Explicit quality measures are developed in advance of the assessment, in contrast to implicit quality assessment that is based on the subjective evaluation of the assessor.[20] The best of the explicit measures are evidence-based, validated, and have been found to be reliable.[19] When a priori assessment measures have not been developed, implicit measures may be used. This type of assessment is based on personal experience or expert judgment.[20] For example, a physician or therapist may be asked to review a patient's care to determine if the care is "good enough."[19]

For certain medical specialties and medical conditions, process and outcome measures have been well-defined. Quality of emergency department care for acute myocardial infarction can be measured by examining the administration of β-blockers and aspirin or by the information derived from an electrocardiogram.[22] For cardiac conditions such as this, outcomes can be measured by mortality. Acute myocardial infarction care shows the ideal relationship between process measures and outcomes measures because there is strong evidence to show that the measured processes have a direct impact on the outcome (death) in question.[23] Few hand surgery or therapy procedures have such well-defined and proved measures, because mortality is usually not a dominant outcome. This makes measuring the quality of hand surgery and therapy much more difficult to assess.

Thinking back to the three domains of quality measurement, it is difficult to say if any one is better than the other for measuring surgical quality. Structural measures, such as hospital or surgeon procedure volume, are easy to obtain, but the value of volume to evaluate quality over a range of procedure has been debated.[24–27] A hospital or a surgeon who perform a large number of a surgical procedure may be shown to have lower mortality and morbidity for this procedure. The good report card given to the high-volume hospitals or surgeons may be caused by other variables, however, such as disease case-mix or intangible factors that may not be entirely attributed to the hospitals and the surgeons. Additionally, structural measures are generally not easily manipulated (eg, to test the effect of volume on outcomes in a clinical trial study design).[28] This makes evaluation of the relationship between structure and outcomes difficult.

Process measures, such as prophylactic antibiotic administration for patients having total joint arthroplasty, are already being used in some surgical quality initiatives.[29,30] Because most process measures are performed by the surgeon or therapist directly, or under his or her direct supervision, they are considered as "fair" quality measures compared with structural measures, which are often outside of surgeons' or therapists' control.[28] Process measures are very procedure-specific, however, and may even be patient-specific. This means that a large number of process measures need to be developed and validated to cover the range of surgical procedures. Finally, process measures may be related to preoperative care rather than actual surgical or postoperative care.[31]

In surgery, outcomes draw the most attention because the end-result is what is important to the surgical patient. Measuring surgical outcomes, however, can be very difficult. Many initiatives that measure surgical quality have used morbidity and mortality as outcome indicators.[32] This is an attractive measure because morbidity and mortality are easily defined and can be obtained from already existing administrative data. Mortality is only relevant, however, for certain high-risk procedures. Unplanned reoperation has been suggested as a possible outcomes measure;[33] like morbidity and mortality, it is easy to define and can be obtained from pre-existing data. A 2007 study in the Netherlands found that 70% of reoperations were caused by errors in surgical technique, making it ideal to measure quality.[33] Unfortunately, from a quality measurement standpoint, reoperation happens relatively infrequently, making it less than ideal for low-volume procedures.[33]

The use of outcome measures is further complicated by the need for careful case-mix adjustment.[31] This avoids "punishing" hospitals and surgeons who take on more complex cases that naturally may have poorer outcomes. Case-mix adjustment, however, is not an exact science. There are multiple methodologies for case-mix adjustment and the use of these different methods can potentially provide differing results.[34] Case-mix adjustment is further complicated by the fact that there is insufficient evidence as to what specific prognostic factors actually govern different outcomes or treatment needs.

Despite these difficulties, surgical quality initiatives do exist. One of the largest is the Veterans Affairs (VA) National Surgical Quality Improvement Program (NSQIP). Established in 1994, NSQIP supplies almost constant feedback, in the form of rankings and outcomes, to VA medical centers on major operations in nine surgical specialties.[35] This feedback allows individual hospitals to monitor their own quality and see how they compare with other VA medical centers. The initiative was originally designed to assess surgical outcomes. The act of measuring and examining the provided feedback, however, induced behavioral changes that resulted in a 27% decrease in 30-day mortality in the first 5 years of the program.[35] In 1998, NSQIP began its private sector initiative, providing feedback on general and vascular surgery to participating academic medical centers and community hospitals.[36]

Accurate measuring of surgical quality has many potential benefits. The first and most obvious is the improvement of the field. Patients stand to benefit from more than just better quality of care. As health care in general becomes more consumer-focused, patients want to make more of their own health care decisions. An excellent field for patients to do this is surgery. Surgical procedures are often planned in advance, giving patients sufficient time to compare different surgeons and hospitals. Furthermore, because surgery is often a one-time event, with patients often returning to their previous physicians for management, patients are willing to travel farther than they would for medical treatment.[32]

MEASURING QUALITY IN HAND SURGERY

The application of quality measures developed for other surgical fields presents a problem for hand surgery. The standard measure for most surgical quality initiatives is mortality. Mortality in hand surgery is less than 1%,[37] however, so it is not a useful outcome indicator. Measuring process and structure is no different for hand surgery than for any other surgical specialty. Process measures that indicate the quality of preoperative care are useful, but do not actually measure the quality of hand surgery performed, in particular the performance of the hand surgery and the level of expertise by the surgeon. Structure measures, such as volume, are of limited use because of many other factors that determine the referral patterns. Structural factors, such as surgeon subspecialty training or therapist certification, have the potential to be predictors of good surgical outcomes.[28] In a very specialized field like hand surgery, this may be an important quality indicator as indicated by the rigor of the training path.

Hand surgery and therapy are unique in that injuries and disabilities of the hand can have substantial impact on patients' quality of life. In lieu of functional outcome measures, such as grip strength or range of motion, patient-rated outcomes have been intensely studied in this specialty.[38] Patient-rated questionnaires, such as the Michigan Hand Outcomes Questionnaire[39,40] or the Disabilities of the Arm, Shoulder and Hand,[41] allow patients themselves to report their own level of functional disability.

APPLICATIONS OF QUALITY DATA
Report Cards

The VA's experience with NSQIP has repeatedly shown that simply providing feedback can promote significant improvements on outcomes indicators, in this case 30-day mortality rates.[42] More often, however, quality data are used to compare entities. The Healthcare Effectiveness

Data and Information Set collects data on 71 measures over eight domains to compare health plans and hospitals.[43] Mostly process and structure measures are used, with patient satisfaction being the only outcome measure. These measures have been criticized for imprecise data quality and poor translation to actual quality of practice.[19,44] Despite the shortcomings, these data are used by many organizations to produce report cards detailing hospital performance on certain surgical procedures. This allows consumers to select where they would like to have their surgery, based on the previous performance of these hospitals.

By far the most popular procedure ranked is coronary artery bypass graft (CABG) surgery. As report cards go, this is an ideal procedure. It is performed frequently at many hospitals and lends itself to the use of mortality as an outcome measure.[45] New York was the first state to begin publicly reporting hospital CABG data in 1990, and currently seven other states regularly publish these data.[45,46] These data are almost exclusively derived from hospital discharge reports and are generally limited to procedure volume and mortality.[46] Private companies also have joined the report card game. Currently, such companies as Health Grades provide for-fee report cards on hospitals, by condition or procedure. These companies rely on Medicare data and report on a wide range of diagnoses, although their coverage of surgical procedure is somewhat lacking. They use a star system (1, 3, or 5 stars, with 5 being the best), rather than reporting actual data, which may be easier for consumers to understand, but can compromise accuracy. Krumholz and colleagues[47] compared Health Grades' ratings with more traditional quality measures, also taken from Medicare data. They found that although the ratings could distinguish between aggregate performance groups, Health Grades' ratings were of no use when comparing individual hospitals.[47] Finally, popular press has begun ranking hospitals. The US News and World Report publishes an annual issue devoted to listing America's best hospitals in 17 specialties using Medicare data and physician surveys. Report cards and national rankings are not solely an American phenomenon. Canada, Great Britain, and Australia all have extensive systems of reporting health care performance.[48–50]

Although these report cards and popular press rankings are aimed at consumers, and are not as rigorous as traditional quality improvement initiatives, they are nonetheless important. As American medicine becomes more consumer-driven, patients take more responsibility in both choosing and paying for their health care. Report cards and rankings provide the transparency that consumers demand. But there is some indication that patients either are not aware of or do not use these reports.[51] Additionally, there are questions regarding their accuracy.[47] Given the push toward more transparency in medical care, the prominence of hospital report cards can only grow.

Even more controversial are physician report cards. Several states publicly publish CABG performance data on individual cardiac surgeons, sometimes including mortality rates. Understandably, this makes many surgeons uncomfortable. These report cards can have unintended consequences. A 1996 survey of cardiovascular surgeons in Pennsylvania found that most surgeons reported that since the commencement of the state's individual surgeon reporting system, they had become less willing to perform CABG on severely ill patients.[52] Perhaps most troubling are consumer ratings of physicians. Zagat, known best for their restaurant guides, has joined forces with an insurance company to provide an interface that allows patients to rate their physicians based on trust, availability, communication, and office environment.[53] Although Zagat's officials freely admit that the ratings are not scientific and reflect patient experience and not quality of care,[53] there is a risk that those reading the reviews may not take this into consideration.

Obviously, no surgeon or hospital wants to provide poor-quality care. Some may believe that the public reporting of quality measures may stimulate improvement among low-performing hospitals. Health care payors have developed ways further to reward quality. Currently, most programs focus on rewarding good performance with monetary bonuses, but there are plans in the works to penalize poor-performing centers by also withholding a percentage of reimbursements.[29]

Centers of Excellence

One of the most basic uses of quality data is the centers of excellence model. In these programs, hospitals that have the best results for a particular procedure are identified and patients are steered toward these centers. Payors do this by limiting payment to only certain high-performing hospitals or by paying for a greater percentage of care at these centers as compared with lower-scoring hospitals.[31] Centers of excellence programs can be based on pre-existing data, such as surgical volume and mortality, making them relatively easy and inexpensive to set up.[31] These data, however, might not be the best predictors of outcomes.[26,27] Access is another problem with the centers of excellence model. Hospitals that are identified as high-quality are not evenly distributed across the country. Payors may have little power to steer patients toward these hospitals if they are not nearby.[54]

Pay-For-Participation

The centers of excellence model does not provide direct monetary incentives to high-performing hospitals, but instead rewards them with more patients. One of the newest incentive schemes, pay-for-participation, does provide monetary incentives, but does so using different standards. In these programs, incentives are given for participation in quality measurement, regardless of actual quality.[31] This is consistent with the philosophy of continuous quality improvement. Pay-for-participation programs create procedure-specific patient outcomes registries. These registries provide regular feedback to hospitals and to individual surgeons and allow for collaboration between hospitals. Meetings are regularly held for participants to discuss performance and brainstorm ways to improve quality. Increased quality is judged collectively, not based on individual hospital or surgeon performance. This structure is the same as that used by the VA for its NSQIP program, which has been very effective in improving performance on surgical outcome measures.[35]

One of the hallmarks of pay-for-participation programs is the lack of public reporting.[31] Because the information is designed to be used by hospitals and surgeons, very specific types of indicators are measured that may not translate well to public report cards. This makes pay-for-participation programs popular among surgeons, but also reduces public support for the programs.[31] The major downfall is that pay-for-participation programs are expensive and complicated to set up. Infrastructure has to be in place for data collection. Every site needs at least one data abstractor and high-level officials need to meet regularly. Their acceptance by surgeons and their ability to improve quality, however, may outweigh these initial costs. The attraction with this model is that the quality can be improved through collective efforts, rather than creating a tier system in which only the top-performing centers are rewarded, whereas the low-performing centers continue to languish at the bottom of the quality spectrum.

Pay-For-Performance

Pay-for-performance takes cues from both the centers of excellence model and pay-for-participation. Simply put, hospitals that score high on selected quality measures are rewarded with a monetary bonus, or likewise, low-scoring centers

are penalized a portion of their reimbursement.[31] When process measures are used as a proxy for quality, pay-for-performance programs have been quite successful in improving adherence to the measured processes.[31] These processes, however, may not be measuring actual surgical care. Despite the potential monetary gain (or threat of monetary loss), pay-for-performance initiatives offer very little in the way of outside motivation. The incentives are often quite low, possibly too low to entice participation, especially for low-performing centers where substantial change and large cost expenditure for infrastructural improvement may be necessary to receive these meager rewards.[55]

The first major, nation-wide pay-for-performance initiative was instituted by the Centers for Medicare and Medicaid Services (CMS) and piloted in 2003. The program uses a classic pay-for-performance model. Core performance measures were developed in such areas as acute myocardial infarction, CABG, heart failure, community-acquired pneumonia, and hip and knee replacement.[29] Quality in these areas was based almost exclusively on process measures. Hospitals report their compliance with the performance measures and CMS then ranks the hospitals based on this performance.[29] These rankings are published on the Internet, and used to distribute incentives and assess penalties. Hospitals that fall in the top 10% receive a 2% bonus on their Medicare payments. Hospitals in the next 10% receive a 1% bonus, and those who round out the top 50% receive recognition for their quality but no monetary reward. Finally, hospitals that have not met minimum performance levels are penalized as much as 2% of their Medicare reimbursements.[29]

There have been some complaints that these measures do not accurately indicate quality of care.[56] In addition, participating institutions need to hire staff to monitor these metrics, often costing more than the potential incentives provided. These complaints are not unique to the CMS program and could be made of any pay-for-performance initiative, yet new programs continue to launch. Consumers continue to demand transparency, payors continue to push for lowered costs, and everyone continues to clamor for higher quality. Stuck in the middle are surgeons, says Dr. Tom Russell, Executive Director of the American College of Surgeons, who feel besieged by these new demands.[57] The quality initiative, however, as presented in the pay-for-performance system developed by CMS, is here to stay.

Hybrid Programs

In 2000, 160 private- and public-sector employers who purchase health care for 34 million people formed the Leapfrog Group.[54] The goals of this group are to reduce preventable medical mistakes; encourage public reporting of quality and outcomes data; reward doctors and hospitals for quality, safety, and affordability; and help consumers make smart health care decisions.[58] A multidisciplinary team identified "leaps" that, when implemented, result in higher health care value, lower costs coupled with higher quality.[54] The four leaps are (1) computerized physician order entry, (2) evidence-based hospital referral, (3) ICU physician staffing, and (4) the Leapfrog safe practice score. The main activity of the Leapfrog Group is an online, voluntary hospital survey. Recently, the Leapfrog Group has introduced a hospital rewards program, based on quality and safety, which provides incentives for both participation and excellence.

The Leapfrog Group is an innovative initiative with the potential to have a great impact on the practice of medicine. The group has a large membership, clear goals, and national recognition. The number of compliant hospitals has doubled for some leaps and several members have been successful in using the leaps to make consumers more value-conscious when choosing a health care provider.[54] The impact has not been as large, however, as it could be potentially. Too few hospitals have opted to participate in the survey and some purchaser-members have been reluctant to use the survey's results to guide their health care purchasing decisions (eg, limiting employees' choices to only high-scoring hospitals).[54] The Leapfrog Group is continuing to expand their program, maintaining their innovative position by assisting large payors in leveraging their buying power to demand changes in payment, decreased costs, the adoption of quality measures, and an overall increase in health care value.

Final Thoughts on Quality Data Applications

Many quality workgroups have organized an effort to steer national dialogs regarding quality-of-care initiatives. As one of these groups, the IOM has issued design principles for pay-for-performance programs, including the use of reliable measures, fostering coordination of care and the rewarding of data collection (**Box 1**).[59] Pay-for-performance programs are seen by many as being the wave of the future, despite there being little evidence that any one program produces superior quality measurement over another.[31]

Often, the question of which model is best is situational. Measuring the quality of risky, uncommon procedures, such as pancreatic resection and esophagectomy, is best done using the centers of excellence model.[31] Pay-for-performance initiatives are best for improving compliance with underused processes of care that are linked to surgical outcomes by a high level of evidence, like venous thromboembolism prophylaxis for high-risk patients.[31] They are not without their flaws. Rosenthal and colleagues[55] examined three preventative care process measures in two pay-for-performance initiatives. They found that practices with the lowest compliance at baseline showed the most improvement.[55] These were not, however, the centers that reaped the most rewards. Practices that had the highest baseline compliance received over 75% of the incentives, although they showed little to no improvement.[55] Despite improving to a much greater degree, the low-baseline practices were not able to reach the payment threshold and were not rewarded for their efforts. This could discourage participation and quality improvement for centers that need it the most. Additionally, centers with low baseline compliance are often centers with less resources.[60] Pay-for-performance initiatives

---

Box 1
Institute of Medicine design principals for pay-for-performance and its implementation

- Use performance measures that reliably define good care and optimal health outcomes
- Reward care that is of high clinical quality, patient-centered, and efficient
- Reward significant provider improvement as well as achievement of excellence
- Foster care coordination among providers
- Reward data collection and reporting functions and encourage adoption of improved information technologies
- Report provider achievement in ways that are both meaningful and understandable to consumers
- Develop performance measures and structure rewards to maximize participation of all providers over time
- Be fiscally responsible
- Implement in deliberately planned phases, evaluate progress, and learn from experience in each phase

From Institute of Medicine of the National Academies. Rewarding provider performance: aligning incentives in Medicare. Report Brief 2006; with permission. Copyright © 2006, National Academies Press, Washington, DC.

that penalize centers that already struggle with a lack of resources, many of whom care for underserved populations, have the potential further to perpetuate health disparities.

Pay-for-participation initiatives avoid this problem by rewarding all providers equally, providing the best potential for overall improvement of surgical quality.[31] This encourages all providers to participate in quality measurement initiatives, regardless of baseline performance. Critics may worry that being rewarded solely for participation may not result in improved performance, but NSQIP has indicated that simply measuring performance can provide better results.[28,35] There are additional benefits. Because there is no need to rank large groups of providers or to provide broad generalizations, these programs can identify procedure-specific processes that are related to important surgical outcomes, rather than being limited to high-volume or high-risk procedures.[31] This makes pay-for-participation useful for all surgical specialties. There are substantial monetary and time-commitment barriers to initiating a pay-for-participation program, but the investment of money pays off in the potential to reduce negative outcomes of all procedures, which can raise the overall value of surgical care.

IMPLICATIONS FOR HAND SURGERY AND THERAPY

The future of health care quality measurement is in no way certain. Surgical societies, such as the American College of Surgeons, American Academy of Orthopedic Surgeons, and the American Society of Plastic Surgeons, are all participating in some way in the quality improvement movement.[10,57,61] Hand surgeons have a duty and an interest to participate in these societies' quality improvement initiatives. The development of accurate quality matrices that are specific to hand surgery is of the utmost importance, ultimately rewarding those who participate in these quality initiatives. Hand surgeons and therapists cannot stand by and hope that the right measures and programs appear. They need to work to make changes and take the future of hand surgery quality into their own hands.

REFERENCES

1. Kaiser health tracking poll: election 2008. Menlo Park (CA): The Henry J. Kaiser Family Foundation; 2007.
2. Blendon RJ, Altman DE, Benson JM, et al. Health care in the 2004 presidential election. N Engl J Med 2004;351(13):1314–22.
3. Health care and the Democratic presidential campaign: CBS News; September 17, 2007.
4. Kaiser Family Foundation poll. Storrs, CT: Roper Center for Public Opinion Research; 2007.
5. National health expenditure accounts: 2006 highlights. Available at: http://www.cms.hhs.gov/NationalHealthExpendData/downloads/highlights.pdf. Accessed March 3, 2008.
6. The World Health Report 2000. Health systems: improving performance. Available at: http://www.who.int/whr/2000/en/whr00_en.pdf. Accessed March 3, 2008.
7. Catlin A, Cowan C, Hartman M, et al. National health spending in 2006: a year of change for prescription drugs. Health Aff 2008;27(1):14–29.
8. Reinhardt UE. The Swiss health system: regulated competition without managed care. JAMA 2004; 292(10):1227–31.
9. Bozic KJ, Smith AR, Mauerhan DR. Pay-for-performance in orthopedics: implications for clinical practice. J Arthroplasty 2007;22(6 Suppl 2):8–12.
10. Pierce RG, Bozic KJ, Bradford DS. Pay for performance in orthopaedic surgery. Clin Orthop Relat Res 2007;457:87–95.
11. Chung KC, Rohrich RJ. Measuring surgical quality: is it attainable? Plast Reconstr Surg, in press.
12. Hsiao WC, Braun P, Dunn D, et al. Results and policy implications of the resource-based relative-value study. N Engl J Med 1988;319(13):881–8.
13. Sherrid P. Mismanaged care? US News World Rep 1997;123:57–62.
14. Ghori AK, Chung KC. Market concentration in the healthcare insurance industry has adverse repercussions on patients and physicians. Plast Reconstr Surg 2008;121(6):435e–40e.
15. Institute of Medicine. To err is human: building a safer health system. Available at: http://www.iom.edu/CMS/AboutIOM.aspx. Accessed April 24, 2008.
16. To err is human: building a safer health system. Washington, DC 2000.
17. Crossing the quality chasm: a new health system for the 21st century. Washington, DC: Institute of Medicine; 2001.
18. Blumenthal D. Part 1: quality of care–what is it? N Engl J Med 1996;335(12):891–4.
19. Brook RH, McGlynn EA, Cleary PD. Quality of health care. Part 2: measuring quality of care. N Engl J Med 1996;335(13):966–70.
20. Donabedian A. The quality of care: how can it be assessed? JAMA 1988;260(12):1743–8.
21. Donabedian A. Twenty years of research on the quality of medical care: 1964–1984. Eval Health Prof 1985;8(3):243–65.
22. Glickman SW, Ou FS, DeLong ER, et al. Pay for performance, quality of care, and outcomes in acute myocardial infarction. JAMA 2007;297(21):2373–80.
23. Lambert-Huber DA, Ellerbeck EF, Wallace RG, et al. Quality of care indicators for patients with acute myocardial infarction: pilot validation of the indicators. Clin Perform Qual Health Care 1994;2:219–22.

24. Birkmeyer JD, Siewers AE, Finlayson EVA, et al. Hospital volume and surgical mortality in the United States. N Engl J Med 2002;346:1128–37.

25. Birkmeyer JD, Stukel TA, Siewers AE, et al. Surgeon volume and operative mortality in the United States. N Engl J Med 2003;349:2117–27.

26. Daley J. Invited commentary: quality of care and the volume-outcome relationship. What's next for surgery? Surgery 2002;131(1):16–8.

27. Sheikh K. Reliability of provider volume and outcome associations for healthcare policy. Med Care 2003;41(10):1111–7.

28. Birkmeyer JD, Dimick JB, Birkmeyer NJ. Measuring the quality of surgical care: structure, process, or outcomes? J Am Coll Surg 2004;198(4):626–32.

29. Darr K. The Centers for Medicare and Medicaid Services proposal to pay for performance. Hosp Top 2003;81(2):30–2, Spring.

30. Bhattacharyya T, Hooper DC. Antibiotic dosing before primary hip and knee replacement as a pay-for-performance measure. J Bone Joint Surg Am 2007;89(2):287–91.

31. Birkmeyer NJ, Birkmeyer JD. Strategies for improving surgical quality: should payers reward excellence or effort? N Engl J Med 2006;354(8):864–70.

32. Broder MS, Payne-Simon L, Brook RH. Measures of surgical quality: what will patients know by 2005? J Eval Clin Pract 2005;11(3):209–17.

33. Kroon HM, Breslau PJ, Lardenoye JW. Can the incidence of unplanned reoperations be used as an indicator of quality of care in surgery? Am J Med Qual 2007;22(3):198–202.

34. Glance LG, Dick A, Osler TM, et al. Impact of changing the statistical methodology on hospital and surgeon ranking: the case of the New York State cardiac surgery report card. Med Care 2006;44(4):311–9.

35. Khuri SF, Daley J, Henderson WG. The comparative assessment and improvement of quality of surgical care in the Department of Veterans Affairs. Arch Surg 2002;137(1):20–7.

36. Khuri SF. Safety, quality, and the National Surgical Quality Improvement Program. Am Surg 2006; 72(11):994–8.

37. Bhattacharyya T, Iorio R, Healy WL. Rate of and risk factors for acute inpatient mortality after orthopaedic surgery. J Bone Joint Surg Am 2002;84-A(4):562–72.

38. Chung KC, Burns PB, Davis Sears E. Outcomes research in hand surgery: where have we been and where should we go? J Hand Surg 2006; 31A(8):1373–9.

39. Chung KC, Watt AJ, Kotsis SV, et al. Treatment of unstable distal radial fractures with the volar locking plating system. J Bone Joint Surg 2006;88A(12): 2687–94.

40. Chung KC, Kotsis SV, Kim HM. A prospective outcomes study of Swanson metacarpophalangeal joint arthroplasty for the rheumatoid hand. J Hand Surg 2004;29A(4):646–53.

41. Beaton DE, Katz JN, Fossel AH, et al. Measuring the whole or the parts? Validity, reliability, and responsiveness of the disabilities of the arm, shoulder and hand outcome measure in different regions of the upper extremity. J Hand Ther 2001;14(2): 128–46.

42. Khuri SF. The NSQIP: a new frontier in surgery. Surgery 2005;138(5):837–43.

43. National Committee for Quality Assurance. What is HEDIS? Available at: http://www.ncqa.org/tabid/187/Default.aspx. Accessed March 18, 2008.

44. Pawlson LG, Scholle SH, Powers A. Comparison of administrative-only versus administrative plus chart review data for reporting HEDIS hybrid measures. Am J Manag Care 2007;13(10):553–8.

45. Steinbrook R. Public report cards: cardiac surgery and beyond. N Engl J Med 2006;355(18):1847–9.

46. Hospitals: how safe?. Available at: http://www.consumerreports.org/cro/health-fitness/health-care/hospitals-how-safe-103/hospital-report-cards/. Accessed April 8, 2008.

47. Krumholz HM, Rathore SS, Chen J, et al. Evaluation of a consumer-oriented internet health care report card: the risk of quality ratings based on mortality data. JAMA 2002;287(10):1277–87.

48. Australian Medical Association. AMA public hospital report card 2007.

49. Shojania KG, Forster AJ. Hospital mortality: when failure is not a good measure of success. Can Med Assoc J 2008;179(2):153–7.

50. Zamvar V. Reporting systems for cardiac surgery. BMJ 2004;329(7463):413–4.

51. Schneider EC, Epstein AM. Use of public performance reports: a survey of patients undergoing cardiac surgery. JAMA 1998;279(20):1638–42.

52. Schneider EC, Epstein AM. Influence of cardiac-surgery performance reports on referral practices and access to care: a survey of cardiovascular specialists. N Engl J Med 1996;335(4):251–6.

53. Gupta S. Rating your doctor. Time New York 2008; 171:62.

54. Galvin RS, Delbanco S, Milstein A, et al. Has the leapfrog group had an impact on the health care market? Health Aff (Millwood) 2005; 24(1):228–33.

55. Rosenthal MB, Frank RG, Li Z, et al. Early experience with pay-for-performance: from concept to practice. JAMA 2005;294(14):1788–93.

56. Werner RM, Bradlow ET. Relationship between Medicare's hospital compare performance measures and mortality rates. JAMA 2006;296(22): 2694–702.

57. Russell TR. The future of surgical reimbursement: quality care, pay for performance, and outcome measures. Am J Surg 2006;191(3):301–4.

58. The Leapfrog Groups for Patient Safety. Available at: http://www.leapfroggroup.org/. Accessed April 25, 2008.

59. Report brief. Rewarding provider performance: aligning incentives in Medicare. Washington (DC): Institute of Medicine; 2006.

60. Rosenthal MB, Dudley RA. Pay-for-performance: will the latest payment trend improve care? JAMA 2007; 297(7):740–4.

61. Hunter JG. Appropriate prophylactic antibiotic use in plastic surgery: the time has come. Plast Reconstr Surg 2007;120(6):1732–4.

Integrating Patient Values into Evidence-Based Practice: Effective Communication for Shared Decision-Making

Ana-Maria Vranceanu, PhD[a], Cynthia Cooper, MFA, MA, OTR/L, CHT[b],
David Ring, MD, PhD[a],*

KEYWORDS

- Patient centered • Evidence based
- Shared decision-making

Increasing data suggest that the traditional clinician-centered or disease-focused, biomedical approach to illness is less effective than a biopsychosocial, evidence-based, patient-centered approach to illness, particularly for chronic pain conditions.[1–3] In contrast to the traditional biomedical model of illness (which reduces every illness to a pathophysiologic disease process), a biopsychosocial approach to illness accounts for the complex interaction among biologic, psychologic, social, and behavioral factors.[2] Evidence-based practice (EBP) integrates the best available scientific evidence with individual clinical expertise and patient preferences.[4] Patient-centered care (PCC) is respectful of and responsive to individual patient preferences, needs, and values[5] and customizes treatment recommendations on the basis of informed, shared decision-making (SDM), development of patient knowledge, enhancement of skills needed for self-management of illness, and preventive behaviors.[6]

In the biopsychosocial illness framework, the goals of EBP and PCC are (1) to provide treatment that is both consistent with the best available scientific evidence and compatible with the patient's values and life context; (2) to optimize wellness, function, and quality of life; and (3) to encourage the most positive, optimistic, practical, enabling, cost- and resource-effective, and empowering illness concepts consistent with the best available scientific evidence. Incorporation of EBP, biopsychosocial conceptualizations, and PCC requires that health providers are familiar with current best evidence and can communicate this knowledge to patients in a manner that respects the patient's values and fosters a good health provider–patient relationship.

This article distinguishes PCC from more traditional and outdated medical decision-making models; illustrates the complexity of illness behavior with a patient example; delves into the communication issues raised by this complexity, thereby demonstrating how best evidence can sometimes run counter to biases and intuition; provides a summary of evidence that PCC positively affects outcomes; and explores how the SDM approach along with cultivation of good communication skills can facilitate EBP.

TRADITIONAL MODELS OF MEDICAL DECISION-MAKING
The Paternalistic Model

The paternalistic model of medical decision-making was the most prevalent approach to treatment within North America before 1980. In this

[a] Orthopedic Hand and Upper Extremity Services, Department of Orthopedic Surgery, Massachusetts General Hospital, Yawkey 2100, 55 Fruit Street, Boston, MA 02114, USA
[b] Scottsdale Healthcare, Medical Plaza IV, 10200 North 92nd Street, Suite 100, Scottsdale, AZ 85260, USA
* Corresponding author.
E-mail address: dring@partners.org (D. Ring).

Hand Clin 25 (2009) 83–96
doi:10.1016/j.hcl.2008.09.003

model the health provider assumes the dominant role and the patient is passive. Two key assumptions underlie the difference in power between patient and health provider in the paternalistic model: that there is a single, best treatment for a particular condition; and that only the health provider has knowledge of this best treatment. The exchange of information is one-way (from health provider to patient) and deals only with biomedical issues.[6] There is no input from the patient.[6]

In the paternalistic decision-making framework the patient is granted the sick role by the provider,[7] and is excused from social, work, and family obligations, while focusing all their energy on "getting well," seeking expert help and complying with the medical regimen. The health provider assumes the expert role, as a "guardian of the patient's interests."[8]

This model has lost favor because there is rarely a single best treatment for a given condition. There are usually several options, each with advantages and disadvantages, benefits and risks. Because the patient has to live with the consequences of the decision, the health provider may not be in the best position to evaluate the cost benefit of the available options.[9,10]

The Health Provider-As-Agent Model

In the health provider-as-agent model, the health provider chooses what he or she believes the patient would elect if the patient had their knowledge. In contrast to the paternalistic model where the decision is based solely on biomedical information, in the health provider-as-agent model an attempt is made to account for the patient's preferences; however, knowledge and information remain the province of the health provider alone. The critique of this model[11,12] is that it is not possible for the health provider fully and accurately to understand the patient's preferences without gathering patient feedback. Research indicates that when health providers infer patients' preferences they are often wrong.[13,14]

The Informed Decision-Making Model

In the informed decision-making model the patient is vested with decision-making and considered to know best how a particular treatment might affect him or her. In this model the patient learns about the risks, benefits, and effectiveness of the alternative treatment options from the health provider and makes a decision that fits his or her preferences.[15] Although some research has shown that older patients and patients with less education prefer less involvement in the decision-making,[16] perhaps this response depends on how the

question is asked. Hanson[17] suggests asking "Do you know your physician to make decisions knowing what is important to you, or without knowing what is important to you," rather than "Who do you want to make the decision about your treatment."

The Shared-Decision Model

According to Charles and coworkers,[6] the SDM model is based on several concepts. First, decision-making involves at least two participants, the health provider and the patient, but may also involve family members, relatives, and friends and multiple health providers. This increases the complexity of the process. Communication is particularly important in this context because variations in opinion may be confusing and stressful for the patient and treatment team. For example, a specialist physician's advice to a patient that the discomfort from lateral epicondylosis does not reflect injury and that remaining active in painful activities will not prevent resolution of the illness may run counter to the primary care provider's recommendation to rest the elbow and avoid pain. These variations in opinion (the so-called "art of medicine") are unavoidable, and may increase the patient's confusion and uncertainty.

The second concept is that all parties (the health providers and the patient and his or her supporters) take steps to participate in the process of decision-making. Research has identified variations in patient comfort with sharing their opinions and participating in the decision-making process. Further, there is some research evidence that often patients' expressed preferences for sharing opinions and participating in the decision-making process do not always correspond with what actually happens (ie, patients often shy away from participating and instead let the health care provider take the lead). This occurs because of several patient characteristics, including personality style, contextual factors, social desirability, and cohort effects.[14] These findings emphasize the importance of exploring a patient's background and developing a strong patient–health provider relationship that allows the patient to become comfortable in the sharing process. For a patient, SDM means that she or he must be willing to engage in the decision-making, disclose preferences, ask questions, weigh and evaluate treatment alternatives, and formulate a treatment choice. This is a problem-solving task that is complex and goes beyond simple information transfer. In the shared-decision model, both parties adopt complementary roles, participate, and are satisfied with their level of involvement.

The third concept is that information sharing is requisite to the shared-decision model. Patients may bring in information from other sources, including acquaintances, media, and other health providers. The provider brings an honest interest in helping the patient, an individualized comfort, and preference for a particular treatment. Instead of the patient bringing the values and the health provider bringing the information, the patient and the health provider both bring information and values. The sharing process is individualized and dynamic.

Lastly, a shared treatment decision is made, to which health providers and patients and supporters agree. The shared decision is both a process (involving complementary roles and exchange of information) and an outcome: the decision. The decision may be agreement on a treatment plan, but may also be to suspend a decision or even to disagree, in which case the patient likely seeks additional health provider opinions. Agreement may not indicate that both parties are convinced that they have elected the best treatment; agreement means only that all parties endorse it as the treatment to implement. The health provider, for example, may believe that a patient should hold off on surgery until he or she is feeling less vulnerable and desperate, but he or she may agree to endorse the patient's decision to proceed with surgery as part of a negotiated agreement in which the patient is informed that there are risks, including persistent symptoms, but the patient's preferences are also valued and accounted for. This characteristic helps distinguish the SDM model from the paternalistic and informed models, where decision-making and ultimate responsibility for the decision are clearly vested with the health provider and patient, respectively, whether or not the opposite party accepts the decision. Research suggests that patient participation in decision-making results in greater patient satisfaction, improved outcomes, and acceptance and adherence to treatments.[18–20]

Patient-Centered Care

SDM and PCC are often used interchangeably in the literature, but some believe that SDM is just one aspect of PCC, which goes beyond the decision and includes the context of illness, the treatment process, and patient–health provider interaction. Over the last decade there has been a strong move toward a patient-centered rather than clinician-centered approach to medical care. This approach is consistent with SDM, and implies shared power and responsibility within the patient–health provider relationship. This

approach is also consistent with the biopsychosocial model, by accounting for the person within the disease.

Stewart and colleagues[21] provide a framework for PCC to describe six interactive components of the patient-centered process: (1) exploring both the disease and the illness experience (history, physical examination, dimensions of illness, such as feelings, ideas, expectations, functionality); (2) understanding the whole person (life history, personal and developmental issues, family, employment, social support, culture, community, ecosystem); (3) finding common ground (developing realistic treatment goals, problem solving and prioritizing, establishing relationship rules and boundaries); (4) incorporating health promotion (eg, health enhancement, early identification, complication reduction); (5) enhancing the patient-provider relationship (compassion, power, healing, transference-countertranference, self-awareness); and (6) being realistic (teamwork, time and timing, wise use of resources).

PATIENT EXAMPLE

Sue is a 41-year-old woman who presents to a hand surgeon with complaints of right lateral elbow pain for 5 months. Sue is trying to start a family and is worried that this elbow pain will keep her from being a good parent. She feels incapable of holding a child in her arms. Her sister had a similar problem and had surgery after several unsuccessful corticosteroid injections, followed by an MRI that was interpreted as showing a "muscle tear." Sue is wary of surgery, but wonders if an MRI will show a tear in her arm that needs surgery.

The Evidence

One conception or summation of the best available scientific evidence regarding Sue's lateral epicondylosis is as follows: (1) it is a benign, age-related, self-limited, degenerative enthesopathy of middle age;[22] (2) corticosteroid injections are no more effective than placebo anesthetic injection;[22–24] (3) there is no evidence that the MRI appearance of lateral epicondylosis or the presence of a defect in the extensor carpi radialis brevis origin affects prognosis;[21] and (4) disability associated with chronic pain correlates with psychologic distress (depression and anxiety), ineffective coping skills (catastrophizing), and heightened illness concern.[25–27]

The Patient's Goals

Under the traditional biomedical illness framework, Sue's goal might be interpreted as being, "to cure my pain." Under the biopsychosocial model, Sue's goal might be seen more broadly, inclusively, and realistically as "to be at ease and confident about my plans to have a child." Both Sue and her health providers are at risk of directing too much attention at an indirect and potentially unattainable goal (complete pain relief), when a more meaningful and attainable goal is at hand: "a restored sense of well-being."

The Biomedical Clinician-Centered Approach to Illness

Under a biomedical (disease-centered), clinician-centered approach to Sue's illness, one can assume that Sue's concerns will all be addressed by a cure of the disease. The clinician prescribes a treatment or diagnostic test intuitively, according to their training, tradition, and bias rather than the best scientific evidence. They then adopt a progressive or algorithmic approach leading to additional treatments based on failure of prior treatments to achieve cure and findings on diagnostic tests.

The impact of this approach on Sue's illness is that what might be conceived of as an extremely common, self-limiting, benign enthesopathy of middle age without effective treatment (a "rite of passage" of human development, so to speak) is transformed (medicalized) into a disease that requires treatment. Moreover, the psychosocial behavioral factors of her illness may be exacerbated by this approach: an opportunity to enhance adaptation, resiliency, peace of mind, and other aspects of wellness is missed; ineffective biomedical approaches to illness are condoned and reinforced, thereby medicalizing the problem and decreasing self-efficacy; and a real or perceived lack of empathy and communication leads to decreased patient satisfaction and adherence to recommendations, not to mention increased medicolegal risks.

Health providers are aware of the limitations of modern medical science, and the consequent "art of medicine" that is practiced; however, clinicians are rarely explicit or mindful about what it is that they are doing when they manage illness beyond the limits of science. By science is meant concepts based on reproducible hypothesis testing; science is knowledge of what will happen (how to manipulate the environment) because experiments have been done and objective reproducible observations have been made. Beyond the limits of science (objective testing) illness concepts are chosen: where the evidence ends are only beliefs or hypotheses. There is a risk that the illness concepts chosen actually exacerbate

the illness by reinforcing illness behavior. For instance, when a health provider voices a belief that a given illness is caused by "overuse," the patient may limit his or her activities unnecessarily. The patient may become less able to do things (more disabled) simply by virtue of the illness concept that is promoted. Illness concepts may lead to serial treatment interventions, which in a surgeon's practice tend to become increasingly invasive and risky. Treatment failures can be both disheartening and medicalizing: "what are we going to do next?"

A Patient-Centered, Evidence-Based, Biopsychosocial Approach to Illness

The authors favor an approach to illness that is based on the best scientific evidence. Such an approach stems from an open discussion of the limitations of modern medicine and the selective use of diagnostic tests and specific treatments, while promoting the most hopeful, positive, adaptive, optimistic, practical, safe, and resourceful illness concepts. Most importantly, the authors favor an approach that addresses the patients' understanding of their illness. This approach allows one to account for the complex biopsychosocial aspects of illness rather than attempting to reduce each illness to a pathophysiologic disease process as is typical of the biomedical approach to illness.

It is important to identify and address sources of distress, social issues, and behavioral issues. Sources of distress tend to fall into one of three categories: (1) catastrophizing (the ineffective coping skill of expecting the worst or interpreting the situation in the worst possible way); (2) depressed mood; and (3) health anxiety or heightened illness concern (the sense that one has a serious illness that persists despite reassurance to the contrary). Examples of social issues include job dissatisfaction or burnout and troubled family situations. The behavioral issues are reflected in habits or intuitive responses to illness (eg, pain avoidant behavior, or a tendency to adopt the sick role).

Having taken this broader view of illness, the health provider and patient should then agree on appropriate goals. Returning to the example of Sue, she and her health providers must be willing to place hope in the many aspects of illness management and temper focus on a cure, because one is not as readily and predictably available as might be wished or imagined. Better goals are (1) maximizing the ability to care for a child; (2) greater peace of mind and confidence; and (3) improved comfort.

The patient-centered approach implies collaboration and agreement on a plan for management.

To temper unrealistic expectations and disproportionate emphasis on the biologic aspects of the illness appropriately, there should be an agreement on the role of diagnostic tests, which are best used to address very specific diagnostic questions that can identify treatment targets that change management based on established treatment effectiveness. It is important to emphasize the value of time as a diagnostic test, because many musculoskeletal conditions are both puzzling and transient.

Likewise, there should be agreement on treatments and an honesty and openness about their roles. For instance, one can be open about which treatments are specific (eg, release of the transverse carpal ligament for carpal tunnel syndrome) and which are nonspecific (eg, pain medication). One thing that patients often misinterpret or misunderstand is the distinction between palliative and potentially curative treatments. For instance, corticosteroid injection for osteoarthritis is a palliative treatment, but without explicitly stating this patients may expect a cure and be needlessly disappointed.

Finally, the patient and health provider should both agree to address all aspects of the illness and all possibilities for increasing wellness, including psychosocial behavioral issues. In a multidisciplinary, team approach, this means that every team member's input is valued and considered.

THE ISSUES RAISED BY EVIDENCE-BASED MEDICINE

Health providers who look to science to help ensure that their approach is as accurate and as free from bias as possible (EBP) face several dilemmas in trying to build and maintain a mutually respectful, empathic relationship with individual patients. Best evidence regarding how to handle diagnostic uncertainty, interpretation of diagnostic tests, descriptions and conceptions of illness, the psychosocial aspects of illness, and what constitutes effective treatment, may be counterintuitive and contrary to the patient's and even the health provider's bias. For these reasons, the SDM model is ideal and good communication skills are paramount.

Diagnostic uncertainty is common in the hand and arm, particularly with respect to pain. Uncertainty and lack of control can be distressing for both the patient and the health provider and it is tempting to place hope in diagnostic testing; however, tests are not perfect and their use for screening various diagnoses should be considered carefully. In a setting of diagnostic uncertainty, the prevalence of a specific disease in the population of patients being tested is very low. When likelihood of a disease is low, the impact of false-positive tests is greater. This is captured in statistical diagnostic performance characteristics, such as prevalence-adjusted positive and negative predictive values, and likelihood ratios. Consider the example of a "suspected scaphoid fracture." Even when using a diagnostic test that is 90% sensitive and specific, the fact that only 1 in 10 or 20 patients with a suspected scaphoid fracture has a true fracture means that a "positive" test corresponds with a true fracture less than half the time.[28] The bottom line is that there is substantial risk of overdiagnosis and overtreatment in the setting of diagnostic uncertainty.

Another issue is the incomplete correlation between findings on diagnostic tests and symptoms. For example, radiographic signs of arthrosis have limited correlation with pain complaints. As another example, 50% of normal asymptomatic wrists have a ganglion cyst detected on MRI.[29] If one combines the potential for overdiagnosis in the setting of diagnostic uncertainly with the limited correlation between diagnostic test results and illness, it becomes clear that diagnostic tests must be used with great care.

Psychologists emphasize the emotive power of words, and the relative emotive power of many English-language words has been studied scientifically.[30] It is important to choose words and illness concepts carefully. One example of a particularly poor choice of words is the indiscriminant use of the word "tear" in orthopedic surgery.[28] The word "tear" implies acute traumatic injury, and damage that may require repair. There are times when this is appropriate, such as a tear of the sagittal band or terminal extensor tendon. Use of the word "tear" to describe degenerative lesions or defects of the rotator cuff, extensor carpi radialis brevis origin, or the triangular fibrocartilage complex may not accurately represent the disease process, however, because many of the defects that occur as a part of these illnesses are not caused by acute trauma and do not need to be healed or repaired.

Returning to Sue, ordering an MRI and being labeled as having a "tear" is likely to be very unsettling, and there is no evidence that this finding will improve the management of her illness. It can be very difficult to communicate to Sue why a specific test should not be obtained, however, when this runs counter to her bias and intuition. Careful choice of words and illness concepts are very important aspects of medical communication.

Many health providers are not mindful of the fact that a large number of diagnoses are illness constructs rather than objectively verifiable pathophysiologic disease processes. Examples include fibromyalgia, chronic fatigue syndrome, repetitive strain injury, chronic regional pain syndrome, radial tunnel syndrome, pronator syndrome, and electrodiagnostically normal carpal tunnel syndrome. Regardless of ones' feelings about the value of these diagnoses, it must be acknowledged that they cannot be verified or falsified with reproducible objective testing and they are not strictly scientific; they are best considered as social constructs, which are terms "invented" or "constructed" by a culture or by a society, and existing because people agree to behave as if they exist.[31,32] Furthermore, although one can debate the usefulness of these illness constructs, there is no debate about their potential to do harm by increasing illness and illness behavior. Many of these concepts are by nature negative, implicating use of the arm or environmental exposures without adequate evidence, or medicalizing common symptoms or normal human development. In Australia, the demonization of occupational hand use and the medicalization of nonspecific activity-related arm pains in the illness construct "repetitive strain injury" led to epidemic illness and disability that reduced greatly when the social situation changed and the diagnosis became not compensable.[33]

The normal function of the human mind as documented by psychologic science has substantial effect on illness behavior. The human mind tends toward black and white thinking (dichotomizing), whereas most diseases and illness occur on a continuous spectrum. This, along with a tendency for health providers and patients to conceive of illness in mechanical, fixable terms, may raise unrealistic expectations and misconceptions. Finally, there is a tendency toward magical thinking, entertaining anything imaginable as possible. Although these aspects of the normal functioning of the human mind have a notable influence on illness behavior, consideration and discussion of the psychosocial and behavioral facets of illness is largely stigmatized in society; the typical patient conceives of the mental aspect of illness as separated and distinct from the physical aspect of illness and often feels offended by discussion of the cognitive, emotional, social, and behavioral aspects of illness (eg, "Are you saying it's all in my head?"). A biopsychosocial behavioral approach to illness requires good communication skills. In communicating with Sue, it is important to be mindful of these aspects of human intuition, thinking, and decision-making.

Perhaps the most important issues raised by EBM are those related to treatment. Much of what patients and surgeons believe is the result of their individual experience (anecdote) rather than scientific investigation. Science has shown the importance of questioning individual experience. If Sue reports relief from a corticosteroid injection for her lateral epicondylosis, she may be experiencing the placebo effect (an important aspect of human psychology that results in real or perceived improvement because of her belief that the injection will help); regression to the mean (the fact that all illnesses wax and wane in symptom severity and she may have received an injection at the peak and by regression gone to a better symptom level, unrelated to any influence of the injection itself); and the normal self-limiting course of the disease (the illness would have improved with or without the injection). Science has not identified a specific effective treatment for lateral epicondylosis, but this must be communicated to Sue without taking away her hope, most or all of which may have been placed on a medical or surgical cure.

The SDM process involves communication of the best evidence regarding the risks and benefits and advantages and disadvantages of various treatments. Although sometimes overlooked in a resource-rich setting, it is also important to consider appropriate use of resources (eg, financial impact) because these are not unlimited and must be shared. Finally, although there is strong and growing evidence that such issues as secondary gain (when a patient stands to benefit from the illness and disability), depression, posttraumatic stress, catastrophizing, and other ineffective coping skills, and health anxiety or heightened illness concern exacerbate disability and illness behavior, it is difficult to put this evidence into practice in modern medical settings. EBP requires open and effective communication of the complex biopsychosocial behavioral nature of illness, something that may be more easily accomplished in a multidisciplinary setting that includes behavioral medicine specialists, nonoperative musculoskeletal providers, and occupational and physical therapists.

OPTIMIZING COMMUNICATION IN EVIDENCE-BASED PRACTICE AND SHARED DECISION-MAKING
Barriers to Evidence-Based Practice

Patients and health providers approach treatment with different agendas and expectations for treatment. Understanding the biases and agendas of all involved parties and resolving discrepancies with effective communication is an important aspect of patient-centered, evidence-based management.

The patient's agenda

Patients approach treatment with a set of expectations and beliefs about illness (some of which are misconceptions) and treatment that are shaped by personal experiences, stories from acquaintances, and cultural and societal factors. Painful illnesses, such as Sue's lateral epicondylosis, are particularly prone to misconceptions. These misconceptions are the crux of the contextual acceptance and commitment therapy for pain management, which has been recently coined by McCracken.[34]

A very common misconception about pain is that it always indicates harm. Patients often measure improvement based on their pain level. Sue may say that she is getting worse after an episode of intense pain, or after a day of painful typing. In addition, patients often present with the expectation that pain is easily diagnosable and treatable: the "quick fix" or "miracle cure," a concept that marketing of medical care seems to exacerbate or reinforce. Patients may also approach treatment in a passive, effortless way, and might not see that they have a role and responsibility in addressing their illness. So-called "doctor-shopping" (frequently changing doctors) may be a consequence of the belief that "a good doctor will take my pain away."

Patients often assume that without pain control the underlying disease will get worse. This natural assumption is often confirmed by experience. For example, removal of a painful, rupturing appendix can be lifesaving. In the arm, neglected painful infections can be limb-threatening or life-threatening. In the context of most chronic pains, however, attempts to limit pain can increase illness. Attempts to control pain often include extended rest, avoidance of activity, time off from work, invasive procedures, and the use of medication. When these strategies do reduce pain they do not necessarily improve physical and social functioning or overall health. By focusing all efforts on achieving pain control, life is disrupted and time that was spent engaging in activities that give meaning to life, such as social relations, hobbies, or work, are replaced with medical visits, financial burden, social isolation, and distress. The search for pain control to live a good life becomes a paradox. As a society, we engender a strong aversion and fear of pain, which often is worse than the pain itself.[35] Indeed it is often not the pain per se, but rather the fear of pain (or pain and suffering about the pain) that restricts one's life and leads to disability and suffering, similar to depression about depression, anxiety about anxiety, or anger about anger. All of these reactions restrict one's capacity to live a full and satisfying life.

The costs of pain avoidance are well documented in terms of inability to function physically, socially, and emotionally.[34,36,37] Control and avoidance often work in the short-term, because the immediate effect of turning away from an activity that provokes fear is to feel relief from fear. The simple action of taking a pill reduces some of the fear, regardless of its pharmacogenic component, and by this mechanism may alleviate pain. Unfortunately, the long-term consequences of avoidance are deleterious: reducing the big picture of one's life to "pain only."

Often patients can engage in cognitive fusion, a process in which thoughts are blended together with the events they describe or the people who experience them.[38] When Sue imagines that she will not be able to hold a child, even though this is actually not happening, she feels and behaves like it is happening, demonstrating cognitive fusion. When a pain sufferer feels the pain and believes that he or she is becoming paralyzed, losing control, or dying, and fails to recognize that this thought is merely a thought, then the thought gets fused with reality. Sue may have a thought, such as "I can't hold a child without pain so I can't be a good mother" and take it as literally true, which can bring about suffering, attempts to avoid the thought, and avoidance of what might otherwise be meaningful and rewarding activities (ie, motherhood). It is important to help patients understand and recognize not only the content of their thinking, but also the process of their thinking, so that they can have more options. This allows them to choose between acting according to a thought or acting in another way that may yield different and more productive results. For Sue, if she understands that "I can't hold a child" and "I can't be a good mother" are just thoughts, not reality, she can choose perhaps to hold things (including a child) in spite of pain, and be able to search and see that she can be a good mother even though her elbow is painful.

Another aspect of psychology that can create problems includes the human habit of "giving reasons" and accepting reasons for their own and others' actions.[38] Shouting at someone when angry, choosing to avoid a situation because of anxiety, staying home when not feeling well are all completely acceptable scenarios that meet with social approval in most circumstances. In the medical realm, fatigue, discouragement, and worry are accepted as good reasons for not engaging in a painful activity. For Sue, avoiding painful activities is accepted and may also be rewarded by family and friends as the "right thing" to do to get better. Humans with chronic pain conditions live their lives according to the explanations they give to themselves. These explanations may also influence how they seek relief or respond to treatment. Understanding these explanations is particularly important in communicating with such patients as Sue. A treatment approach that seeks overt behavior change for pain without considering whether that approach matches the patient's view of his or her problem may yield limited results. For example, prescribing no restrictions in activity to a patient without understanding that patient's view of the pain conditions and activity may be ineffective because the patient may return with increased reasons as to why she or he cannot engage in activities without restrictions.

An important barrier to providing evidence-based treatments to patients is that evidence-based treatment recommendations often do not correspond with and may even conflict with the patient's intuition about what ought to be done. The patient who reports pain and limitation of activity to avoid pain is acting consistently, and this consistency makes good sense to the patient and those around him or her. By the same reasoning, to be suddenly more active without reduction in pain makes no sense to the patient or the people in his or her life. Social influences on expected behavioral consistency over time, across situations, and between speech and action can be very restricting for pain sufferers, particularly when the action that works best for them in the long run contrasts with what they have said or done in the past. If Sue returns to painful activities her pain may be dismissed by family and friends because her change in behavior is deemed inconsistent with true illness. This is representative of some of the very important and underappreciated behavioral aspects of illness.

Messages from media and the Internet are shaping the culture's views on health and wellness. Treatments are perceived as requisite for health. Perfect health is seen not only as attainable, but also as right. Such conditions as arthritis or Sue's lateral epicondylosis, age-related conditions of normal human development, are medicalized and become diseases that need to be cured. This goal to become "cured" and "pain free" is often unattainable, which creates a strong barrier to EBP and SDM.

The health provider's agenda

Hand and arm health providers may lack appreciation for the psychosocial factors impacting patient's lives. They may operate from the biomedical approach viewing pain as black or white, biologic or psychologic. When noticing psychologic issues they may have difficulty communicating the need to address those issues because of the stigmatization of psychologic illness present in society (the sense that psychologic aspects of illness imply "weakness" or lower status), and an unrealistic belief in own abilities to heal (eg, "god syndrome"). Consistent with the biomedical model, health providers may also believe that any psychosocial issues will resolve once the physical treatment is successfully implemented.

In addition, health providers tend to use intuition and clinical experience rather than EBP.[39,40] Their own experiences, habits, beliefs and attitudes, clinic's norms, and social factors have greater influence on treatment than the scientific literature.

Stress can also influence decision-making. The patient's distress in the form of depression and anxiety, catastrophizing, and heightened illness concern can be contagious (a process known to psychologists as "countertransference"). Health providers may be more inclined to believe that a patient's pathophysiology is more severe in the face of more intense reports of pain intensity and disability, even when the clinical evidence does not support this line of thinking.[41,42]

Health providers feel pressured for time and many believe that they do not have sufficient time to understand and address their patient's goals and agendas in detail. Treating patients with complex pain conditions that are diffuse, vague, and ambiguous, with disproportionate reports of pain intensity and disability can also be very frustrating to health providers.[43,44]

Noncompliance, unrealistic expectations, uncomfortable and inappropriate demands, and personality clashes can threaten EPB and SDM.[44] Often, surgeons feel pressured to provide specific treatments to avoid upsetting the patient and the referral source. Finally, commercial influences may also impact decision-making.

How Shared Decision-Making can Facilitate Evidence-Based Practice

The dilemma of EBP is that the best evidence is often at odds with a health provider's or patient's intuition, preconceptions, expectations, or prior experiences. For instance, although Level 1 evidence suggests that corticosteroid injection is not effective for lateral epicondylosis, Sue may know someone who had a great result from injection, she may have confidence about injections according to what she has read or heard from other doctors, and it may fit her preconception and intuition that there is a quick and simple answer to her problem. Although the best scientific evidence certainly is useful and valuable to Sue, she may not be receptive to it if she perceives it as paternalistic and uncaring. The collaborative environment that results from adoption of SDM can help Sue feel more receptive to ideas that are counterintuitive or even unwelcome.

A key element of the shared-decision model is the creation of an atmosphere in which the patient believes that his or her views are valued and needed.[45] Good communication skills are requisite. The health provider should develop the ability to elicit patient goals and preferences to ensure that the options discussed are compatible with the patient's lifestyle and values. It is also important to be able to provide technical information in an unbiased, clear, and simple manner, and to help patients conceptualize the process of weighing risks and benefits. Research suggests that detailed health information reduces uncertainty and increases reassurance while aiding decision-making.[12]

The patient–health provider relationship is a "partnership in patient care."[46] This implies that the relationship between the health provider and patient is consensual rather than obligatory. The provider may communicate with authority while not being authoritarian. The patient may pose questions, offer alternatives, look for other opinions, or select a different provider. In the shared-decision model, health providers assume several simultaneous roles: information gatherer; recorder; interpreter; coach (prompting patients to ask certain questions); advisor (advising patients about the advantages and disadvantages of various options); negotiator (advocating on the patient's behalf); and caretaker (supporting and reinforcing the patient's decision).

There must be respect and trust between both parties. If the patient's request is incompatible with what the health professional believes is in his or her best interest or conflicts with the professional's personal beliefs and standards, the provider should not compromise his or her medical, ethical, or personal standards. For instance, if Sue insists that corticosteroid injection is the only way to treat her elbow pain, her health provider may disagree on the basis of his or her interpretation of the best evidence and specific to Sue's situation. Although one hopes that Sue would consider her health provider's opinion carefully, she may not be prepared to consider alternative illness concepts, and may instead disregard her health provider's preference and continue to insist that injection is the only option. Under the shared-decision model, the health provider should not allow a patient's inflexible view to dictate the course of treatment. Rather, the health provider may suggest that patient should seek a second opinion, try

conservative treatments, or re-evaluate the situation at a different point in time. Encouraging and conveying appropriate positive expectations by good communication skills can be very helpful in this process and can allow for disagreement without compromising the relationship.

The health-patient interaction is a process that involves "windows of opportunity."[47] Health providers should listen for and acknowledge changes in a patient's appearance, emotion, posture, or voice. This change tends to occur in the middle of the clinical visit. Picking up on this change and using it to help broach a discussion of potentially sensitive aspects of the illness may be of value in understanding a patient's life context and other aspects of illness behaviors, preferences, and style of decision-making. For instance, health providers may find it helpful to inquire with compassion and empathy about suspected causal relationships and other patient assumptions to be sure that they are based on best evidence. There should be open discussion when the patient may stand to benefit from their illness (eg, litigation, worker's compensation, disability, narcotic addiction, and other areas of secondary gain). Perhaps most difficult, it is ideal to be able to discuss a patient's uneasiness, difficulty being reassured, or depressed mood.

The health providers should be able to introduce options and share their own opinions, beliefs, and preferences without imposing their own values. Distinguishing the caregiver's view from the patient's view[48,49] and clarifying roles in a constructive and empathic manner is important. The health provider may experience frustration when coalitions occur and the interaction seems adversarial (eg, patient and family against health provider). Staying attuned to this frustration and refraining from blaming the patient is a key. It is important to know when to end the conversation while conveying empathy and formulating goals for the next visit.

Communication Skills: The Key to Effective Evidence-Based Practice and Shared Decision-Making

The health provider–patient relationship is one of the most important predictors of patient satisfaction, adherence to medical treatment, and overall treatment success.[50] Health providers whose communication styles are less dominant receive higher satisfaction ratings than health providers who communicate in a paternalistic or authoritative manner.[20]

Health providers should be mindful of biases, both their own and those of the patient. Patients and health providers may have their own theories about what is best based on scientific research (best evidence), or reports from family, friends, or media. Both providers and patients may become victims of the self-serving bias, whereby information that disproves one's beliefs is dismissed with minimal consideration, and information that is consistent with a belief is given priority. Sue may be focused on her view of pain as meaning damage, and may not be able to shift her focus toward accepting that that is not the case with her lateral elbow pain. She may keep bringing up that her elbow hurts and she cannot use it, while dismissing the fact that the pain does not mean damage. The health provider may be particularly focused on the message she or he delivers, and fail to account for the patient's agenda. This may cause conflict and interfere with the decision-making process.

It is also beneficial to be aware of the emotive power of words, and their strong impact on a patient's response to treatment and coping styles.[51] Words with relatively negative connotations, such as "tear," "injury," or "overuse," are remembered more than words with a positive connotation. When health providers use the word "tear," they may mean to imply the normal defects or developments of aging, or a benign condition that does not require treatment; however, to the patient the word "tear" implies injury, damage, and the need for treatment or repair. It is important for health providers to choose their words carefully, and use alternative words with a more accepted neutral or positive message to replace words with a more negative message (eg, benign defect instead of tear). When such words are not available, a thorough explanation of word choice is merited. In a similar vein, it is important to avoid medicalization of pain conditions that are a part of normal human development whether permanent and incurable (eg, arthritis) or temporary and self-limiting (lateral epicondylitis). Furthermore, clarification that many conditions are genetic or developmental and not the result of "overuse" or "injury" can relieve the guilt and regret that patients often feel when they have pain associated with activity.

The key elements of good communication are trust, empathy, and confidence in the health care provider. Patients must perceive that their health care provider listens, understands, and appreciates their suffering.[52] Before beginning to address a challenging patient situation, it is helpful to take a few moments mentally to settle, to try taking a few deep breaths, and reach a clear state of mind. These steps help cultivate mindfulness, which includes being nonjudgmental and present in the moment.[53] The health provider should also

try to listen without interruption at the beginning of the session; to summarize the patient's statements using the patient's words; to legitimize the patient's concerns by repeating them or restating them; and to express empathy[47] ("this must be difficult for you," "wow") and normalize the situation ("most people in your situation would react the same way"). When providers listen, they elicit their patients' stories. By telling their stories, patients find words that help them manage their situation, which fosters control over the chaos of illness. The provider who takes interest in the meaning of patients' stories is practicing narrative medicine. This humanistic approach is exemplified by the practice of medicine that includes reflection, professionalism, trustworthiness, and empathy.[54]

To experience empathy, the provider must enter the patient's subjective world and try to comprehend what it is like to be in that person's situation.[55,56] It is easier to do this (ie, to be empathic) with people who are like ourselves; it is harder to be empathic with people who are different from us,[57] and to do so usually requires emotional labor. Instead of making assumptions about what the patient would like the clinician to address or do, introduce options and follow the patient's preferences. Before addressing difficult issues (eg, divergences between best evidence and patient preconceptions, heightened illness concern, or misconceptions and catastrophizing), it is important to be sure that one has made a "deposit in the patient's emotional bank account." One needs to gain the patient's trust and confidence, and foster in them a benevolent and forgiving attitude before raising potentially contentious or offensive issues.

Patients need to feel that their health care provider has expertise. The health care provider must show confidence in their skills, discuss treating similar patients, provide a thorough explanation of symptoms, and explain the shortcomings of diagnostic and treatment strategies. The health provider should instill and preserve hope: instead of "I don't know what's going on" or "I have nothing to offer you," try "I wish it were as easy as a surgery or medication, but a creative approach that considers all possibilities is effective," or "we have helped many patients in situations similar to yours with a comprehensive team approach." It is also important to acknowledge the stigmatization of the psychologic and sociologic aspects of illness. It can be difficult to discuss uneasiness, health anxiety, and depression without offending. Good communications skills require a constant focus on the positive.

Good communication skills influence treatment acceptance, adherence, and outcome. Patients are more motivated if their provider is enthusiastic and energized; polite and respectful; celebrates gains (even small ones); exhibits friendly or open facial expression; and provides eye contact. Demonstrating integrity, following-up as promised, and returning calls are also important. Using the first visit to develop rapport in some instances may be more fruitful than providing a complete clinical evaluation but not having time to develop that rapport.

Interactions with patients who have prominent psychosocial issues can be frustrating. Patients with certain personality disorders, hostility and anger, or alcohol and drug concerns, patients who have had negative interactions with providers in the past, and patients with limited financial resources (especially in high-stress situations) can be particularly difficult. In such situations the physician-patient relationship and patient participation are even more important than in a typical situation. Taking the time to listen and understand the patient's context and the reasons for his or her behavior or demands may help diminish stress and frustration, while helping to share empathy and an honest desire to help. Lowering one's voice in response to a patient with an aggressive voice, listening attentively with no interruptions, asking permission to examine and share in the conversation are small but powerful accommodations that help greatly in developing the relationship, diffusing anger, and planning accordingly for a shared treatment approach. In particular, requesting permission is a very strong demonstration of respect (eg, "Can we discuss some of the things that are making you feel uneasy?"; "Would you like to hear some of the advantages and disadvantages associated with the test/procedure?"; "This part of the examination can be painful, but it's very important. May I proceed?").

Cooper and others[58,59] provide suggestions for how to navigate communication where patients resist participation in the shared-decision model. In this situation the health provider must refrain from acting as an expert telling the patient what to do; communication requires a two-way conversation. A statement, such as "you should do these exercises," may lead to defensiveness in patients, whereas an open question, such as "what can you do today that you think will make it better?" may help the patient think about their condition in a different way, and one in which they are responsible for recovery. Positive, optimistic language is important. For instance, "even a few minutes of exercise will help" rather than, "it's going to be hard to make time for all these exercises." There may be less resistance to recommendations made for a future visit when saying "you may be ready to try new exercises next week," rather than when

saying "we have to add these new exercises right now." Statements such as "you know your hand better than I do; show me what feels OK for you," rather than "I will teach you how to treat your hand," may reinforce the patient's confidence, and self-efficacy.

Offering choices and having the patients pick among several options may also work well with difficult or resistant patients. For example, instead of "you have to exercise 5 repetitions 5 times a day," try "would you prefer to do 5 reps 5 times a day or 3 reps 10 times a day?" Paradoxical suggestions, such as "going home and exercising every hour would probably be too much trouble," rather than "when you go home you will have to exercise every hour" may be perceived as a challenge that the patient chooses to take on, rather than as a task that he may not want to undertake. Minimizing the directiveness of the health provider is also helpful, because it emphasizes that the patient benefits from doing the work for himself or herself. A statement, such as "it can be extremely helpful to elevate your arm," is better than "I need you to elevate your arm."

Remarks that help the patient envision resumption of important and valued activities may increase confidence and motivation to try. For example, a statement such as "you still can't hold a golf club and I don't know when you will" is negative and uncertain, whereas "in the future, when you are holding your golf club..." shows confidence and empowers the patient to try. Allowing the patient control can build trust and confidence. Instead of telling patients what to do, "I'm going to have you start with this exercise, and do 10 repetitions," ask their opinion: "What do you want to start with? How many repetitions of this exercise do you think you should do?"

THE MULTIDISCIPLINARY TEAM APPROACH TO EVIDENCE-BASED PRACTICE AND PATIENT-CENTERED CARE

Multidisciplinary treatment teams that consider the psychosocial and the biomedical aspects of illness have proved useful in the management of the most common idiopathic pain conditions, including backache and headache,[60–62] and discrete pain conditions, such as arthritis.[63] Although many hand and arm pains are poorly understood and incompletely treatable, and psychosocial factors, such as depression and anxiety, often exacerbate discrete pain conditions, hand surgeons and hand therapists have been slow to implement multidisciplinary treatment teams. Instead, they largely continue to operate under a biomedical model of illness potentially neglecting prominent and treatable psychosocial factors. Despite the support of scientific evidence on the unique contribution of psychologists to the understanding of the multifactorial nature of pain,[64] and recommendations from governing bodies, such as the Joint Commission on the Accreditation of Health Care and the Commission on the Accreditation of Rehabilitation Facilities, and several professional organizations (American Pain Society, American Academy of Neurology), the psychologist's role is underappreciated, seen as potentially offensive, and is currently undervalued by patients, health providers, and insurers. A multidisciplinary approach to treatment of hand and arm pain conditions is consistent with EBP and fits well within the patient-centered model of medical decision-making. Having more than one listener allows the patient to feel cared for because there is a team of doctors and therapists, rather than one, attending to the pain concern. This may increase the patient's confidence that nothing is overlooked and all possibilities for increasing wellness are considered.

The gap between the utility and the use of a multidisciplinary treatment team is at least in part caused by the difficulty communicating the value of a biopsychosocial approach to illness to patients and their health providers. This gap itself represents an example of the need for good communication in the integration and practice of evidence-based medicine and PCC. The quest for best evidence necessitates input that is more multilayered and more complex, reflecting less tissue-focused specificity and greater richness and breadth than the historically valued reductionistic approach associated with the medical model. Treating illness, not just disease, requires that various aspects of the patient's situation be addressed, even though these factors may be ambiguous or contradictory. It requires more involvement and results in more empowerment of patients. This is best implemented by a multidisciplinary team through treatment processes that value and embrace effective communication skills.

REFERENCES

1. Jensen MP, Romano JM, Turner JA, et al. Patient beliefs predict patient functioning: further support for a cognitive-behavioral model of pain. Pain 1999;81:95–104.
2. Turk DC, Gatchel R. Approaches to pain management: a practitioner's handbook. 2nd edition. NY: The Guilford Press; 1999. 360.
3. Turk DC, Okifunji A, Sinclair JD, et al. Treatment for fibromyalgia: clinical and statistical significance. Arthritis Care Res 1988;11:186–95.
4. Sackett DL. Evidence based medicine: what it is and what it isn't. BMJ 1996;312:71–2.
5. Stewart M. Towards a global definition of patient centered care. BMJ 2001;322(7284):444–5.
6. Charles C, Gafni A, Whelan T. Decision-making in the physician-patient encounter: revisiting the shared treatment decision-making model. Soc Sci Med 1999;49:651–61.
7. Parson T. The social system. New York: The Free Press; 1951.
8. Emmanuel EE, Emmanuel EL. Four models of the physician-patient relationship. JAMA 1992;267:2221–6.
9. Eddy D. Anatomy of a decision. JAMA 1990;263: 441–3.
10. Lomas J, Lavis J. Guidelines in the mist. Paper presented at: Centre for Health Economics and Policy Analysis, 1996; McMaster University, Hamilton, Ontario.
11. Evans R. Strained mercy: the economics of Canadian health care. Toronto: Butterworths; 1984.
12. Mooney G, Ryan M. Agency in health care: getting beyond first principles. J Health Econ 1993;12:12–5.
13. Strull WM, Lo B, Charles G. Do patients want to participate in medical decision making? JAMA 1984; 152:19–90.
14. Ryan M. The economic theory of agency in health care: lessons from non-economists for economists. Paper presented at: Health Economics Research Unit Discussion Paper, 1992; University of Aberdeen, Scotland.
15. Hurley J, Birch S, Eyeles J. Information, efficiency and decentralization within health care systems. In: CHEPA Working Papers 92-21. Ontario (Canada): McMaster University; 1992.
16. Swenson SL, Buell S, Zettler P, et al. Patient-centered communication: patients really prefer it? J Gen Intern Med 2004;19:1069–79.
17. Hanson J. Shared decision making: have we missed the obvious? Arch Intern Med 2008;168:1368–79.
18. Gwyn R, Elwyn G. When is a shared decision not (quite) a shared decision? Negotiating preferences in a general practice encounter. Soc Sci Med 1999;49(4):437–47.
19. Elwyn G, Edwards A, Hood K, et al. Achieving involvement: process outcomes from a cluster randomized trial of shared decision making skills development and use of risk communication aids in general practice. Fam Pract 1991;21(4):337–46.
20. Kaplan SH, Greenfield S, Gandek B, et al. Characteristics of physicians with participatory decision-making styles. Ann Intern Med 1996;124(5):497–504.
21. Stewart M, Brown JB, Weston WW, et al. Patient-centered medicine: transforming the clinical method. Sage Publications, Inc.; 1995. 267.
22. Boyer MI, Hastings H. Lateral tennis elbow: is there any science out there? J Shoulder Elbow Surg 1999; 8(5):481–91.

23. Altay T, Gunal I, Ozturk H. Local injection treatment for lateral epicondylitis. Clin Orthop Relat Res 2002;398:127–30.

24. Lindenhovius A, Hanket M, Gilligan BP, et al. Injection of dexamethasone versus placebo for lateral elbow pain: a prospective, double-blind, randomized clinical trial. J Hand Surg 2008;33:909–19.

25. Price R, Sinclair H, Heinrich I, et al. Local injection treatment of tennis elbow: hydrocortisone, triamcinolone and lignocaine compared. Br J Rheumatol 1991;30(1):39–44.

26. Ring D, Kadzielski J, Malhotra L, et al. Psychological factors in idiopathic arm pain. Journal of Bone and Joint Surgery 2005;87:374–80.

27. Vranceanu AM, Safren S, Ring D. Psychiatric illness predicts disability and idiopathic versus discrete hand and arm pain. Clin Orthop Relat Res 2008; 466:2820–6.

28. Adey L, Souer JL, Lozano-Calderon S, et al. Computed tomography of suspected scaphoid fractures. J Hand Surg 2007;32(1):61–6.

29. Lowden CM, Attiah M, Garvin G, et al. The prevalence of wrist ganglia in an asymptomatic population: magnetic resonance evaluation. J Hand Surg 2005;30(3):302–6.

30. Bradley MM, Lang PJ. Affective norms for English words (ANEW): stimuli, instruction manual and affective ratings. Technical report C-1. Gainesville (FL): The Center for Research in Psychophysiology, University of Florida; 1999.

31. Williams GR, Rockwood CJ, Bigliani LU, et al. Rotator cuff tears: why do we repair them? Journal of Bone and Joint Surgery 2004;86:2764–76.

32. Putnam M. Linking aging theory with disability models: increasing the potential to explore aging to physical impairment. Gerontologist 2002;42: 799–806.

33. Reilly P. Repetitive strain injury: from Australia to UK. J Psychosom Res 1995;39(6):783–8.

34. McCracken L. Contextual cognitive-behavioral therapy for chronic pain. Seattle (WA): International Association for the Study of Pain; 2005.

35. Crombez G, Vlaeyen J, Heuts PH, et al. Pain-related fear is more disabling than pain itself: evidence on the role of pain related fear in chronic back pain disability. Pain 1999;80:329–39.

36. Bortz WM. The disuse syndrome. West J Med 1984; 141:691–4.

37. McCracken LM, Spertus I, Janeck AS. Behavioral dimensions of adjustment in persons with chronic pain: pain-related anxiety and acceptance. Pain 1999;80:283–9.

38. Hayes SC, Sthrosal K, Wilson KG. Acceptance and commitment therapy: an experiential approach to behavioral change. New York: Guilford Press; 1999a.

39. Bhandari M. Evidence-based orthopaedics: a paradigm shift. Clin Orthop Relat Res 2003;413:9–10.

40. Schünemann HJ, Bone L. Evidence-based orthopaedics: a primer. Clin Orthop Relat Res 2003;413: 117–32.

41. Doornberg JN, Ring D, Malhotra L, et al. Pain dominates measurements of elbow function and health status. Journal of Bone and Joint Surgery 2005; 87(8):1725–35.

42. Fernandez E, Turk DC. Sensory and affective components of pain: separation and synthesis. Psychol Bull 1992;112:205–17.

43. Schwenk T. Physician and patient determinants of difficult physician-patient relationships. J Fam Pract 1989;28:59–63.

44. Hahn R, Thompson K, Wills TA, et al. The difficult doctor–patient relationship: somatization, personality and psychopathology. J Clin Epidemiol 1994;47: 647–57.

45. Brody D. The patient's role in clinical decision making. Ann Intern Med 1980;93:718–22.

46. Quill T. Partnerships in patient care: a contractual approach. Ann Intern Med 1983;98(2):228–34.

47. Branck WT, Malik T. Using windows of opportunity in brief interviews to understand patient concerns. JAMA 1993;269:1667–8.

48. Mattingly C. The narrative nature of clinical reasoning. Am J Occup Ther 1991;45:998–1010.

49. Mattingly C. Clinical reasoning. In: Mattingly C, Fleming M, editors. Clinical reasoning: forms of inquirey in a therapeutic practice. Philadelphia: F.A. Davis Press; 1999.

50. Platt FW, Gordon GH. Field guide to the difficult patient interview. Philadelphia: Lippincott Williams & Wilkins; 1999.

51. Lang E, Hatsiopoulou O, Koch T, et al. Can words hurt? Patient-provider interactions during invasive procedures. Pain 2005;114(1,2):303–9.

52. Schofield NG, Green C, Creed F. Communication skills of health-care professionals working in oncology: can they be improved? Eur J Oncol Nursing 2008;12(1):4–13.

53. Pipe TB. Fundamentals of client-therapist rapport. In: Cooper C, editor. Fundamentals of hand therapy: clinical reasoning and treatment guidelines for common diagnoses of the upper extremity. 1st edition. St. Louis (MO): Mosby; 2007.

54. Charon RC. Narrative medicine: a model for empathy, reflection, profession, and trust. JAMA 2001; 286(15):1897–902.

55. Yerxa EJ. Seeking a relevant, ethical, and realistic way of knowing for occupational therapy. Am J Occup Ther 1991;45(3):199–204.

56. Yerxa EJ. Confessions of an occupational therapist who became a detective. Br J Occup Ther 2000; 63(5):192–9.

57. Larson EB, Yao XJ. Clinical empathy as emotional labor in the patient-physician relationship. JAMA 2005;293(9):1100–6.

58. Cooper C, Graff WS, Evarts JL. Psychological techniques to promote patient participation. Poster presented at: American Society of Hand Therapists' Annual Meeting, 2007; Phoenix, AZ.

59. Rosen S. My voice will go with you: the teaching tales of Milton H. New York: Erickson; 1982.

60. Bruce BK, Hooten WM, Rome JD, et al. Chronic pain rehabilitation in chronic headache disorders. Curr Neurol Neurosci Rep 2008;8(2):94–8.

61. Flor H, Fydrich T, Turk DC. Efficacy of multidisciplinary pain treatment centers: a meta-analytic review. Pain 1992;49:221–30.

62. Gatchel RJ, Okifuji A. Evidence-based scientific data documenting the treatment and cost-effectiveness of comprehensive pain programs for chronic non-malignant pain. J Pain 2006;7:779–93.

63. Keefe FJ, Caldwell D, Williams DA, et al. Pain coping skills training in the management of osteoarthritic knee pain: a comparative study. Behav Ther 1990; 21:49–62.

64. Simon E, Folen RA. The role of the psychologist on the multidisciplinary pain management team. Psychology, Research and Practice 2001;32(2): 125–34.

Using an Evidence-Based Approach to Measure Outcomes in Clinical Practice

Joy C. MacDermid, BScPT, PhD[a,b,]*, Ruby Grewal, MD, MSc[c],
Norma J. MacIntyre, PhD[d]

KEYWORDS

- Outcome • Measures • Evaluation • Self-report
- Questionnaires • Evidence-based • Osteoarthritis • Hand

The evidence-based practice approach is made up of five steps:

1. Ask a specific clinical question.
2. Find the best evidence to answer the question.
3. Critically appraise the evidence for its validity and usefulness.
4. Integrate appraisal results with clinical expertise and patient values.
5. Evaluate the outcomes.

Step 5 in the evidence-based practice approach involves evaluating the outcomes of evidence-based decisions in clinical practice. Using the following problem as an example, we can see how to use an evidence-based approach in making decisions about applying evidence on outcome measures to evaluate the status of individual patients.

PROBLEM

Recently, your clinic has experienced a dramatic increase in the number of patients presenting for management of hand osteoarthritis. Some patients are presenting with isolated arthritis of

the first carpometacarpal (CMC-1) joint and others with diffuse involvement of the small joints of the hand. Pain, reduced grip and pinch strength, and inability to perform tasks of daily life are common problems in these patients. For the most part, these are active people, most are female, and many are in the last years of their occupation or are retired but want to participate in a variety of occupational and recreational activities. You have had preliminary discussions with other clinics who agree that hand osteoarthritis is expanding as an area of practice (ie, patients are expecting better functional use of their hands for longer periods of time). You assume that this is partly related to the trend for "healthy aging," but is also related to increased awareness of options for surgical and rehabilitative management as patients are increasingly inquiring about options they learned about on the Internet. You are unsure about specific interventions or the best timing of conservative versus surgical management for this particular population. Given patient expectations and the current state of evidence, you conclude that ongoing measurement of patient-based pain and disability outcomes will be important when

Funded by a New Investigator Award, Canadian Institutes of Health Research.

[a] Hand and Upper Limb Centre Clinical Research Laboratory, St. Joseph's Health Centre, 268 Grosvenor Street, London, Ontario, N6A 3A8, Canada

[b] School of Rehabilitation Science, McMaster University, Institute for Applied Health Sciences, 1400 Main Street West, 4th Floor, Hamilton, Ontario L8S 1C7, Canada

[c] Division of Orthopedic Surgery, University of Western Ontario, Hand and Upper Limb Centre, St Joseph's Health Care, 268 Grosvenor Street, London Ontario, N6A 4L6, Canada

[d] School of Rehabilitation Science, McMaster University, Hamilton, Ontario, Canada

* Corresponding author. School of Rehabilitation Science, LB33, McMaster University, Institute for Applied Health Sciences, Room 429, 1400 Main Street West, 4th Floor, Hamilton, Ontario L8S 1C7, Canada.
E-mail address: macderj@mcmaster.ca (J.C. MacDermid).

making informed program decisions within your clinic and when making treatment decisions with individual patients. Surveying other clinics, you find that some are using the Patient Rated Wrist/Hand Evaluation (PRWHE) (**Fig. 1**), the Australian/Canadian Hand Osteoarthritis Index (AusCan Index), or the Canadian Occupational Performance Measure (COPM) for this clinical population. You are not familiar with any of these measures. You have used the Disability of the Arm, Shoulder and Hand (DASH) questionnaire for some other patient subgroups but wonder if a regional or more specific outcome measure would be best. You would like to choose one or two of these measures for your clinical environment, so you decide to develop a plan for how to incorporate these into your routine management of patients with hand osteoarthritis.

IDENTIFYING THE ATTRIBUTES OF INTEREST IN AN OUTCOME MEASURE

The first step in choosing an outcome measure is deciding what attributes are of clinical interest. The World Health Organization's International Classification of Functioning, Disability and Health is increasingly being used as the conceptual framework for defining health attributes.[1–8] This classification system considers broad constructs from structure to function (activity and participation), while taking into account personal and environmental contextual factors (facilitators and barriers) that mediate the impact disease conditions have on a particular individual. Outcome measures have been developed that provide information regarding a variety of these constructs comprising the International Classification of Functioning, Disability and Health framework.

There is a marked difference between the preferences of clinical researchers/epidemiologists and those of clinicians in their selection of relevant outcome measures. The former have tended to rely primarily on self-report measures, perhaps because these are considered more global and may be easier to administer consistently within the context of clinical trials. Clinicians on the other hand are highly reliant on impairment measures to guide treatment decisions.[9] This is consistent with the biomedical model. The theoretical assumption is that physical impairments lead to functional disability and that, by selecting specific treatment interventions to ameliorate physical impairments, we can restore functional ability. The evidence on physical impairment and functional disability shows a fairly consistent, although moderate, relationship, across most musculoskeletal conditions. Therefore, it is clear that we must measure both

physical impairment and functional disability to fully understand health.

The attributes of interest generated by the clinical encounter above are pain characteristics, grip/pinch strength, and ability to perform tasks of daily life and to participate in recreational activities. As clinicians, we may choose additional attributes of interests that are related to our area of expertise or impairments that we can correct by using the interventions we have to offer. For example, anatomic alignment or thumb stability might be an impairment not specifically identified by the patient, but one we feel contributes to the underlying functional complaints. Similarly, we may know that self-efficacy is highly related to patient's ability to deal with their impairments or to participate in self-management programs. Based on these considerations, we would generate additional attributes of interest and prioritize their measurement so that we can make appropriate decisions regarding the fit of the potential measures and the relative burden they add to clinical care.

In our scenario, we might decide that grip/pinch strength (impairment) and a self-report measure that addresses pain and function (activity/participation) are the attributes of primary interest in our particular clinical environment. Next, we consider basic information on the attributes assessed by available instruments. Grip and pinch strength assess the force voluntarily produced by a patient during active isometric contraction of hand muscles as transmitted through the joints to an external sensor during specific types of grip and pinch. The AusCan Index is a 15-item scale that addresses pain, stiffness, and function. It takes approximately 3 minutes to complete and each item is scored on a five-point Likert scale (zero to four), where the overall or subscale score is expressed as a mean of the items. The PRWHE is also a 15-item scale that takes approximately 3 minutes to complete. There are 5 pain items and 10 function items (6 specific and 4 comparing to usual activity). Items are scored 0 to 10 and 50% of the total score is composed of the pain score (5 items). The other 50% is the disability score (score from 10 items divided by two). The COPM is administered through a semistructured interview process and takes approximately 30 minutes to complete.

SEARCHING FOR OUTCOME MEASURES

Once we determine what instruments or attributes we want to measure, we need more detailed information on validated outcome measures. Searching for literature on outcome measures is more

Name: _____ Date: _____

PATIENT RATED WRIST/HAND EVALUATION

*The questions below will help us understand how much difficulty you have had with your wrist/hand in the past week. You will be describing your **average** wrist symptoms **over the past week** on a scale of 0-10. Please provide an answer for* ALL *questions. If you did not perform an activity, please* ESTIMATE *the pain or difficulty you would expect. If you have **never** performed the activity, you may leave it blank.*

1. PAIN

Rate the average amount of pain in your wrist/hand over the past week by circling the number that best describes your pain on a scale from 0-10. A zero (0) means that you did not have any pain and a ten (10) means that the pain is the worst possible (i.e worst you have ever experienced or that you could not do the activity because of pain).

RATE YOUR PAIN:	None										Worst
At rest	0	1	2	3	4	5	6	7	8	9	10
When doing a task with a repeated wrist/hand movement	0	1	2	3	4	5	6	7	8	9	10
When lifting a heavy object	0	1	2	3	4	5	6	7	8	9	10
When it is at its worst	0	1	2	3	4	5	6	7	8	9	10
How often do you have pain?	0	1	2	3	4	5	6	7	8	9	10
	Never										Always

2. FUNCTION

A. SPECIFIC ACTIVITIES

*Rate the **amount of difficulty** you experienced performing each of the items listed below - over the past week, by circling the number that describes your difficulty on a scale of 0-10. A **zero** (0) means you did not experience any difficulty and a **ten** (10) means it was so difficult you were unable to do it at all.*

	No Difficulty										Unable To Do
Turn a door knob using my affected hand	0	1	2	3	4	5	6	7	8	9	10
Cut meat using a knife in my affected hand	0	1	2	3	4	5	6	7	8	9	10
Fasten buttons on my shirt	0	1	2	3	4	5	6	7	8	9	10
Use my affected hand to push up from a chair	0	1	2	3	4	5	6	7	8	9	10
Carry a 10lb object in my affected hand	0	1	2	3	4	5	6	7	8	9	10
Use bathroom tissue with my affected hand	0	1	2	3	4	5	6	7	8	9	10

B. USUAL ACTIVITIES

*Rate the **amount of difficulty** you experienced performing your **usual** activities in each of the areas listed below, over the past week, by circling the number that best describes your difficulty on a scale of 0-10. By "usual activities", we mean the activities you performed **before** you started having a problem with your wrist/hand. A zero (0) means that you did not experience any difficulty and a **ten** (10) means it was so difficult you were unable to do any of your usual activities.*

Personal care activities (dressing, washing)	0	1	2	3	4	5	6	7	8	9	10
Household work (cleaning, maintenance)	0	1	2	3	4	5	6	7	8	9	10
Work (your job or usual everyday work)	0	1	2	3	4	5	6	7	8	9	10
Recreational activities	0	1	2	3	4	5	6	7	8	9	10

APPEARANCE- OPTIONAL

How important is the appearance of your hand? ▫Very Much ▫•Somewhat ▫ Not at all

Rate how dissatisfied you were with the appearance of your wrist/hand during the past week.

	0	1	2	3	4	5	6	7	8	9	10
	No Dissatisfaction										Complete Dissatisfaction

Any other comments?

Fig. 1. Patient rated wrist/hand evaluation. (*Courtesy of* Joy C. MacDermid, BScPT, PhD, London, ON. Copyright © 2008; used with permission.)

complicated than it is for conventional clinical questions, such as diagnosis, prognosis, or treatment effectiveness. A number of search engines and strategies have focused on how to optimize searches for these classic clinical questions. For example, PubMed uses "Clinical Queries" to assign optimal filters to assist in finding an appropriate subset of information on these specific types of clinical questions. However, no such filter or system exists to help identify all the relevant literature for outcome measures.

Within the scientific literature, evidence on outcome measures exists across a spectrum of study designs. The most common studies investigate psychometric properties of the measures themselves. Any individual research study could focus on a range of psychometric properties: reliability, validity, responsiveness, or translation. Within each of these studies, a variety of subtypes and approaches to analysis exist. Therefore, when we have searched for evidence on outcome measures to conduct systematic reviews, we have tended to use long Boolean search strategies to optimize our retrieval efficiency and effectiveness. Our research strategy tends to take on the generic form of searching for terms that focus on the most common terms/approaches used in psychometric evaluation (*reliability* or *validity* or *responsiveness* or *translation* or *cross-cultural* or *validation* or *factor analysis* or *Rasch* or *item-response*) and the different terms used for outcome measures (*self-report* or *questionnaire* or *survey* or *outcome measure* or *outcome scale*) and the specific content area or instruments of interest (*osteoarthritis* or *hand* or *COPM* or *Canadian Occupational Performance Measure* or *Aus-Can* or *Patient Rated Wrist Hand Evaluation* or *PRWHE* or *DASH*). In using this approach, we were able to identify 27 articles that addressed outcome measures for hand osteoarthritis, most of which were relevant to our question. This was a sufficient number of articles from which to choose a measure and identify comparative data. Thus, at this point we were confident that there would be some measures that had supporting validation work in patients with osteoarthritis affecting the hand.

However, when applying outcome measures to individual patients, clinicians need more than just information on the psychometric properties. Firstly, they need information on how to obtain the instruments, to acquire permission to use them, to administer them, and to score them. To avoid copyright infringement, investigators are often reluctant to include the actual instruments in their published studies. Therefore, obtaining these instruments can be difficult. Using an Internet search engine for the instruments or contacting the developers are two strategies that can be used to obtain this information. In searching for these instruments, we were able to locate a Web site for the AusCan Index (http://www.auscan.org/). From this Web site, we were able to identify an application process for licensing. The AusCan Index has a licensing fee (per user), versions in multiple languages, and a user guide for purchase. Separate agreements need to be completed by each clinician planning to use the AusCan Index. The cost for licensing ongoing use of one particular version of the AusCan Index—the AUSCAN LK 3.1 English for USA Index—for personal noncommercial use and to track the progress of the licensee's own patients in routine clinical practice while those patients remain under the licensee's care, is in three parts:

> AusCan licensing fees for ongoing noncommercial use of the AUSCAN LK 3.1 English for USA Index in their own routine clinical practice: USD$295.00
> One copy of AusCan User Guide III at $60.00 per copy: USD$60.00
> Airmail and handling charges to send the materials to licensee in the United States: USD$40.00

The COPM also was identified on a Web site (http://www.caot.ca/copm/index.htm) that provided an additional description, ordering information (fees associated), and frequently asked questions. The COPM manual/form kit costs USD $52.45 and the COPM Self-Instructional Program Video Kit costs USD $225.45. The PRWHE user manual was also identified using a Google search (http://www.srs-mcmaster.ca/Portals/20/pdf/research_resources/PRWE_PRWHEUserManual_Dec2007.pdf) and is available for free open access.

A third type of information that might be needed to apply outcome measures to individual patients is comparative data. This type of information might be available from normative studies or clinical outcome studies. Normative studies provide data representing the mean level of the attribute in the population, while comparative clinical outcome studies represent the mean outcome score attained from people in similar clinical subgroups, such as individuals with postoperative carpal tunnel syndrome or carpometacarpal osteoarthritis. Data from unaffected individuals provide scores obtained in persons identified as not having the attribute of interest. So, for example, comparative scores from a sample who have recovered from CMC-1 arthroplasty, from an age-matched population sample, and from a sample of older individuals who are known to not have CMC-1 osteoarthritis would represent three different comparative scores.

Clinicians should use standardized, validated, and reliable measures to evaluate their clinical decisions. Before using a measure, it should be screened to confirm that the measures have documented procedures that could be used by others and have been investigated for reliability and validity. Homegrown outcome measures remain popular but have little value because scores for your clinic patients cannot be compared externally and cannot be interpreted by others.

ASSESSING THE VALIDITY OF OUTCOME MEASURES

When evaluating the validity of an outcome measure, information obtained from multiple studies must be considered. Ideally, systematic reviews should be conducted on individual measures or be used to compare measures that look at similar attributes to provide the broad scope of information needed to make decisions about the right tool for different contexts and purposes. Only recently have such systematic reviews started appearing in the literature. There are no "levels of evidence" for individual studies investigating the psychometric properties of outcome measures. Also, individual studies alone provide insufficient information for judging the merits of a specific outcome measure. **Box 1** presents the criteria for judging individual studies that we use when critically appraising these types of studies. The first author of this article (MacDermid) can provide the forms and a guide for completion of this critical appraisal tool. The forms and guide are also published in the textbook *Evidence-based Rehabilitation.*[10] We have used these critical appraisal tools to conduct systematic reviews on the psychometric properties in a variety of outcome measures including shoulder, tennis elbow, shoulder instability, and the neck disability scales.

SELECTING AN OUTCOME MEASURE AMONGST COMPETING CHOICES

When there are multiple measures for attributes of interest, it is necessary to choose between "competing" measures. The first step should be to exclude measures that are not reliable or valid. Studies making head-to-head comparisons of different instruments can be useful to determine if one measure is more valid than the other for the population and purpose of interest. Clinicians should look particularly at responsiveness studies

---

Box 1

Evaluation items for critical appraisal of study design for psychometric articles

Study question

1. Was the relevant background research cited to define what is currently known about the psychometric properties of the measures under study, and the need or potential contributions of the current research question?

Study design

2. Were appropriate inclusion/exclusion criteria defined?
3. Were specific psychometric hypotheses identified?
4. Was an appropriate scope of psychometric properties considered?
5. Was an appropriate sample size used?
6. Was appropriate retention/follow-up obtained? (studies involving retesting or follow-up only)

Measurements

7. Documentation: Were specific descriptions provided or referenced that explain the measures and their correct application/interpretation (to a standard that would allow replication)?
8. Standardized methods: Were administration and application of measurement techniques within the study standardized and did they consider potential sources of error/misinterpretation?

Analyses

9. Were analyses conducted for each specific hypothesis or purpose?
10. Were appropriate statistical tests conducted to obtain point estimates of the psychometric property?
11. Were appropriate ancillary analyses done to describe properties beyond the point estimates (confidence intervals, benchmark comparisons, standard error of measurement/minimum important difference)?

Recommendations

12. Were the conclusions/clinical recommendations supported by the study objectives, analysis and results?

Total score

Percent ([subtotals/24] × 100) based on criteria met from the rating guide and scored as 2, 1, or 0, depending on compliance with standards

This box lists the criteria rating the quality of a study addressing the psychometric properties of an outcome measure. The full form and guide are available from the first author (MacDermid) and are in the textbook *Evidence-based Rehabilitation.*[10]

Courtesy of Joy C. MacDermid, BScPT, PhD, London, ON. Copyright © 2008; used with permission.

that compare each instrument's ability to detect clinical change over time (ie, after treatment) since evaluation of change is the most common purpose for using an outcome measure in clinical practice. In hand surgery and rehabilitation, a number of reliable and valid measures are available. In general, instruments that are anatomically or pathologically specific tend to be more responsive than generic measures.[11,12] Patient-centered measures where the person picks the item (such as the COPM or a Patient-Specific Functional Scale) are also more responsive than generic measures. If instruments are relatively equivalent with respect to measurement properties, then choosing among these involves a number of subjective decisions. Which one is most suitable for the pathologies I see in my practice? Which is easiest to score? What is the cost or training required? How meaningful are the scores? Will my patients accept it? How many measures can I incorporate? What translations are available?

APPLYING OUTCOME MEASURES TO INDIVIDUAL PATIENTS

Many clinicians are reluctant to use self-report measures to make clinical decisions either because they think they are too "soft/subjective" or because they have no intuitive feel for the numbers generated. Clinicians are often surprised to find out that self-report measures may be more reliable than impairment measures, such as strength or radiographic measures. They also forget that over time they have developed an intuitive sense for the clinical meaning of scores from impairment measures. This intuitive sense forms part of their clinical wisdom. Fortunately, we can accelerate the learning curve and make clinical decision-making more evidence-based by using measurement principles to help guide interpretation of self-report scores. In our experience, within 1 to 2 months of consistently using a measure with patients, most clinicians develop some intuitive sense for score meaning (eg, expected levels of disability at various stages of recovery). This enables clinicians to better identify patients who are reporting experiences inconsistent with their stage of recovery or apparent disability.

What Does the Patient's Score Mean?

Methods for defining the meaning of the patient's score include (1) comparing the score to data from uninjured/unaffected individuals or normative data and (2) comparing the score to data obtained from groups with specific problems or levels of disability. These different comparisons provide different perspectives. Data from uninjured/

unaffected individuals tell us what scores might be expected in the absence of pathology. Normative scores provide an estimate of the population mean on a given attribute/measure—usually subdivided on the basis of different demographics, such as age and gender. Outcome studies that provide scores from patients before treatment and across different relevant clinical end points during the recovery process provide useful comparative data with which to "benchmark" individual patient progress. In some cases, this recovery data is presented as growth curves so that clinicians can compare their patient's recovery to usual recovery at different points in time. Ideally, clinicians should have access to all these different forms of comparison data so that reasonable goals can be set and communicated to patients and payers, and recovery and final outcomes can be evaluated in an evidence-based manner.

Many disability questionnaires (like the AusCan, PRWHE and COPM) do not have normative data and assume that no pain and disability would be optimal. In contrast, normative data for the DASH questionnaire are published[13] and presented on the American Academy of Orthopaedic Surgeons' Web site [14] and in the DASH questionnaire user's manual.[15] Comparative scores for different patient populations obtained from studies involving patients with hand osteoarthritis are listed in **Table 1**. In clinical practice, we can compare scores reported for clinical subgroups most similar to our own to indicate an expected level of disability.

How Confident Are We Regarding Individual Patient Scores?

To answer this question, one must know the amount of error associated with each measured value. The standard error of measurement (SEM) reflects measurement error by conveying how much a score is likely to vary with repeated measurements of the same subject. SEM is usually calculated from data available in reliability studies (reliability coefficient and sample variation). Unfortunately, many investigators do not include SEM in their reliability studies, but usually report its components, allowing this value to be calculated.

Although there are several methods for calculating the SEM, a commonly used method is as follows:

$$SEM = \frac{(sample \times standard\ deviation)}{\sqrt{1 - reliability\ coefficient}}$$

When considering a patient's score, it must be appreciated that the measured value is only a representation of the true score and is subject to measurement error. The patient's true score is most likely to lie within a defined confidence interval. Some clinicians use SEM to define their error margins. One SEM is associated with the 68% confidence interval. To obtain higher confidence levels, the SEM can be multiplied by z-values associated with different confidence levels. For example, 1.65 is the z-value associated with the 90% confidence level. This level of confidence is commonly used when making decisions about individual patients because it represents a high level of confidence but is not so rigid that only patients with extreme changes could be judged as improved. The SEM is influenced by the both the reliability of the measurement (represented by the relevant reliability coefficient) and the variability of that population (reflected by the standard deviation). To calculate the approximate SEM with a 90% confidence interval and the minimal detectable change (MDC) for the outcomes of interests (see **Table 1**), we used reliability estimates from the literature, although not specific to hand osteoarthritis, and standard deviations reported for hand osteoarthritis patients.

What Magnitude of Change in Score Indicates that a Patient Has Truly Changed?

When determining whether a patient has changed, we compare scores obtained at two different points in time—each associated with some measurement error. To be confident that we are observing an actual change (beyond that accounted for by error), we need to incorporate an adjustment for this dual source of error. The MDC at a 90% confidence level (MDC_{90}) is obtained as follows:

$$MDC_{90} = \left(Zscore_{90} \text{ or } 1.64 \right) \times \sqrt{2} \times SEM$$

What Magnitude of Change in Score Indicates that the Patient Has Experienced a Clinically Important Difference?

In addition to considering true change, clinicians are interested in determining whether the change experienced by a patient is clinically significant or important. The term *clinically important difference* (CID)[16–19] is often used to describe this quantity. This amount is usually determined by comparing the change in scores on an outcome measure reported in patients who are improved versus the change reported for those who have not improved following an intervention.[18,20] A variety of methods can be used to define these subgroups and choice of methods[18,19,21,22] can affect the estimates. However, a discussion of

this issue is beyond the scope of this article. There is little documentation in hand surgery/hand therapy literature on the CID for different outcome measures. It has been reported that a change of one point is clinically important for the symptom severity scale for carpal tunnel syndrome.[23] Pain scales have been studied for arthritis, including hand osteoarthritis.[24] Here a reduction of one point or a reduction of 15.0% in the numerical rating scale (NRS) for pain (NRS is 0–10) is a CID. A change in NRS score of −2.0 and a percent change score of −33.0% are associated with the concept of being "much better."[24] These values can be considered as the minimum target for therapy or surgical intervention. Ability to make change and CID vary across the spectrum of possible scores. Patients with a high baseline level of pain on the NRS (score >7), who experienced at least a slight improvement had absolute raw and percent changes greater than did patients in the cohort with lower baseline levels of pain (score <4).[25] When faced with patients at the high or low end of the spectrum, we should consider that smaller changes may reflect clinically important differences. We might also need to use alternative instruments that are more responsive to the spectrum of disability we encounter to avoid floor and ceiling effects.

What Amount of Change Is Consistent with the Patient's Goal?

Setting a long-term goal for a patient requires familiarity with the outcome measure of interest and the level of disability consistent with reaching important life outcomes. The level of disability on any measure of interest should reflect the baseline score and the treatment effect size estimated for a particular patient. We can use data from outcome studies or validation studies to provide guidance on these benchmarks. For example, data obtained by Beaton[26] on scores on the DASH questionnaire for working and nonworking patients with upper extremity pathology indicate that the patients who were working had scores in the 20s, whereas the patients who were not working had scores in the 50s. Ideally, the goals set for patients should use principles of clinical measurement. Short-term goals for any outcome measure should exceed the 90% SEM value to ensure that change is beyond measurement error. Long-term goals should be based on the CID, evidence from the literature in terms of the effect size shown for the intervention/outcome measure of interest, and how it relates to life outcomes. Discharge reports can comment on whether the initial pain/disability was consistent with the pathology/comparative scores in the literature

Table 1
Measurement properties of self-report measures in hand osteoarthritis

Properties	Measure Instruments				
	DASH Score	AusCan Index	PRWHE	COPM	
Attributes measured	Function at the personal level (includes pain, symptoms, activity, and participation items)	Pain, stiffness, and function (hand)	Pain and function (hand/wrist) including specific activities and usual activity (participation)	Patients define their occupational performance problems in 3 areas—self-care, productivity, and leisure—during a semistructured interview; patients rate the importance, their current performance, and their satisfaction with performance	
Score range	0–100	0–4	0–100	1–10	
Time to complete	5–7 min	4–7 min[30]	3 min	30 min[31,32]	
Normative values	11 DASH points	Unknown	Unknown	Not applicable	
Reliability coefficients	0.92	0.94 for basal joint arthritis[30]	0.95	0.85	
Standard error of measurement	For basal joint arthritis: 7[29]	For basal joint arthritis: 0.3[29]	For basal joint arthritis: 6[29]	Generic from manual: 2	
90% confidence in a score	11	0.4	10	3	
Minimal detectable change	16	0.6	14	5	
Clinically important difference	~15 DASH points; for distal upper extremity diagnoses: 24[33]	Unknown	12–25; for distal upper extremity diagnoses: 17[33]	Unknown	

| Important clinical benchmarks | Outcomes of 4-corner arthrodesis in wrist osteoarthritis 39 vs. 45 for full arthrodesis

Outcome of Arpe procedure for carpometacarpalosteoarthritis: 2[34]

Change in DASH observed with nasal joint arthritis: 17[35]

Score following arthrodesis of distal interphalangeal joint: 15[36]

Outcome score in proximal row carpectomy (mixed indications): 18[37]

Wrist denervation: 17[38]

Entire flexor carpi radialis tendon harvest for thumb carpometacarpal arthroplasty: 12[39]

Preoperative score of 49 for scaphoid trapezium pyrocarbon implant for osteoarthritis was reduced to 39[40]

Resection arthroplasty of carpometacarpal—abductor pollicis longus group: 20; flexor carpi radialis group: 29[41]

Arthrodesis of osteoarthritic carpometacarpal joint: 32[42]

Carpometacarpal joint arthroplasty (Caffiniere prosthesis): 24[43]

Stabilization of the prearthritic trapeziometacarpal joint using ligament reconstruction: 23[44]

Outcome of tendon interposition arthroplasty: 22[45] | Pretreatment score in 87 women with osteoarthritis: 1.8[31,32]

In community-dwelling elderly with hand problems, from 700 osteoarthritis cases (Genetics of Generalized Osteoarthritis study of familial osteoarthritis) AusCan total 34 of 75; pain 12 of 25; stiffness 2 of 5 (authors did not use recommended scoring)

Outcome score in proximal row carpectomy (mixed indications): 25[37]

Outcome of tendon interposition arthroplasty: 21[45] | Pretreatment score in 87 women with osteoarthritis was 5.2 for performance and 4.8 for satisfaction[31,32]

Actual change reported for patients with hand osteoarthritis undergoing 4 mo of undefined treatment was 1.5 for performance and 2.2 for satisfaction[31,32] |

(continued on next page)

Table 1
(continued)

Properties	Measure Instruments			
	DASH Score	AusCan Index	PRWHE	COPM
Important subgroups		Factors associated with worse scores: older age, female, more carpometacarpal involvement, more distal interphalangeal involvement, more Heberden's nodes[46]		
Other				The most common occupational performance problems identified included opening jars, washing floors, doing up buttons, putting on stockings, carrying groceries, knitting, vacuum cleaning, cutting bread, cross-country skiing (study conducted in Norway), writing, sewing, peeling vegetables[31,32]

We used data from reliability studies on mixed populations of hand-injured patients and standard deviations from papers on hand osteoarthritis[26,29,30,47–49] to calculate standard error of measurement/minimal detectable change. Note: although the AusCan Index should be scored 0 to 4, and subscales should be presented as means, a number of investigators have not followed the recommended scoring algorithm and have just provided a summative or percentage score.

and whether the size of treatment effect achieved was consistent with expectations from current evidence. While this may seem overwhelming, a few properly worded sentences (and a cheat sheet of comparative scores like those provided in **Tables 1** and **2)** are all that is needed.

PLANNING AN OVERALL APPROACH TO MEASURING OUTCOMES IN THE CLINIC

The overall approach involves following 10 steps to identify an appropriate measure:

1. Identify the conceptual framework and/or concepts that are important to measure.
2. Identify a potential list of outcome measures/instruments by searching in textbooks and on line for scientific articles on outcome measures and for articles addressing treatment effectiveness in a similar patient population.
3. Remove any outcome measures that are not standardized, that are clearly not suited to your purpose or situation, or that have been shown to be unreliable or invalid.
4. Critically appraise your potential outcome scale or scales using a standardized process or instrument, or using basic principles to ascertain reliability, validity, and clinical utility (see **Box 1**).
5. Determine whether the instrument you have chosen can evaluate change, predict change, and discriminate in the manner required for your population and purpose.
6. Obtain the measures of interest, and determine the scoring mechanism and any specific instructions on administration (including whether valid translations are available).
7. Identify copyright, reimbursement, and compliance issues.
8. Devise and document a strategy outlining the procedures to be followed when implementing outcome measures into practice (ie, when they will be applied, who will provide them, how/when they will be scored, where the data will be retained, how the data will be used). Make relevant tables of comparison data easily accessible. Ensure that all parties involved participate in devising the implementation strategy and understand their roles.
9. Pilot test one or two instruments for a specified period and re-evaluate the instrument's performance, feasibility, and implementation process.
10. Finalize your choice and a set a time frame to review outcomes data.

IDENTIFYING AND ADDRESSING BARRIERS WHEN IMPLEMENTING THE PLAN

A number of practical issues must be considered when attempting to incorporate new measures into the clinical setting. Expect and prepare for a learning curve. Inadequate preparation inevitably leads to frustration and an inability to use outcome measure scores in making clinical decisions. To facilitate the use of outcome measures, it may be help to (1) employ computerized systems, (2) make paper instruments readily available for use, (3) involve the team in establishing the importance of the measure, (4) provide measures at standardized times, (5) make sure the forms are filled out entirely by the patients, and (6) provide resources/support for scoring.

Although health professionals voice strong support for outcome measures, action is inconsistent with their strong intentions (see the article by MacDermid and Abraham on knowledge translation). Rates of using disability outcome measures are low.[9] Most clinicians still use impairment measures (ie, range of motion, strength, and radiographs) to make treatment or status decisions despite the fairly good evidence that self-report disability scores are better predictors of important outcomes, such as return to work.[27]

The first author (MacDermid) is currently leading a trial comparing different knowledge-translation strategies for increasing clinical use of outcome measures in rehabilitation.[28] While the trial is ongoing, focus groups have been completed to identify barriers and facilitators. In identifying advantages to using outcome measures, clinicians say that outcome measures:

> Facilitate communication with other health professionals/funders
> Improve credibility
> Improve insight into patient perceptions
> Assist in development of realistic goals
> Help focus treatment

The collection and use of outcome measures come with challenges. Clinicians report that outcome measures

> Require additional learning and administration time
> Depend on patient compliance
> Introduce unfamiliar documentation and practices
> Rely on time-consuming score calculations prone to inaccuracy
> Face possible skepticism or lack of understanding from payers
> Add to staff frustration

Table 2
Measurement properties of performance-based impairment and activity limitation measures in hand osteoarthritis

Attribute	Grip Strength: Ability to Exert a Grip Force			Dexterity: Ability to Manipulate Different Sized Objects Quickly (NK Dexterity Test)		
	Grip	Key Pinch	Tripod Pinch	Small Objects	Medium Objects	Large Objects
Time to complete	2–5 min			7–15 min		
Normative values (dominant hand)	50 lb (22 kg)[50a]	11 lb (5 kg)[a]	14 lb (6 kg)[a]	37 s	25 s	39 s
Reliability coefficients (dominant hand) test-retest	0.95[51]	0.98[52]	0.92[53]	0.69	0.72	0.81
SEM	1 kg	0.3 kg	0.6 kg	10 s[b]	5 s[b]	8 s[b]
90% confidence in a score at an instant in time	2 kg	0.5 kg	1 kg	16 s	8 s	13 s
MDC90	3 kg	1 kg	2 kg	23 s	11 s	18 s
Clinically important difference	5 kg for stroke;[54] not known for hand osteoarthritis	Not known for hand osteoarthritis	Not known for hand osteoarthritis	Not determined		
Important clinical benchmarks						
Score for grade 2 osteoarthritis	22 kg		7 kg			
Score for grade 3 osteoarthritis	20 kg		7 kg			
Score for grade 4 osteoarthritis	13 kg		4 kg			
Scores for a recovered ligament reconstruction tendon interposition[29]	21 kg	4 kg	3 kg	55 s	43 s	69 s
Scores for silastic arthroplasty in hand osteoarthritis[55]	18 kg	3 kg	4 kg			

[a] Values vary by age, sex (full details published).[50] These are for females 65 to 69 years old.
[b] For a mixed group of hand pathologies.

Rely on data that may be difficult to collect from some patients (who, for example, may find forms difficult to read)

Can discourage patients if they do not improve

Tend to involve measurement instruments that are too lengthy

Fail in many cases to capture concepts of interest

To help them implement and make best use of outcome measures, clinicians felt they would benefit from:

Computerization

Appropriate studies on outcome measures

Instruments that were easily scored

Having others prepare outcome packages

Administrative staff support

Clear concise instructions

More information on the reliability of outcome measures

Mandates from governing bodies

In our experience, the most useful process to initiate use of an outcome measure is to have the team review their current use and beliefs about outcome measures and then use the process described in this paper to trial one or two new outcome measures. After 1 month, the team can discuss their experiences, compare and contrast the instruments, and clarify barriers to the process. Usually the need, benefit, and motivation for using outcome measures increase during this evaluation period. The process helps define the plan for incorporating and customizing a single or multiple measures into clinical practice to meet the evaluation needs of the team.

In This Case

We asked a group of clinicians from a variety of different clinical settings to review the four scales mentioned in the problem presented in this article. They found the AusCan Index too difficult to score and were concerned about the cost of the start-up and annual license fee. However, they liked having a pain scale because the literature shows pain is an important predictor of function in arthritis. They noted the PRWHE had the same number of items and a pain scale, and they liked the 0 to 10 scaling because that approach is commonly used in practice and is familiar to patients. They also preferred free access. They liked the COPM, but were concerned it might be too time-consuming for their practice. They thought that the Quick DASH questionnaire was good because it had comparative data but were concerned that it

was not validated specifically for hand osteoarthritis and seemed to record lower scores than hand-specific scales, making them question whether the DASH questionnaire would identify all the relevant issues for this patient group (since some of the comparative scores approach normal). However, they also noted that Quick DASH questionnaire would be useful for many patients in the clinic and allow them to evaluate the impact of osteoarthritis at multiple joints. They noted that the DASH/QuickDash could be useful for multiple patient subgroups in their clinic and would allow them to evaluate the impact of osteoarthritis at multiple joints.[29] As a result, they decided to trial the QuickDASH questionnaire and the PRWHE for 1 month and then proceed with one or both on a more consistent basis. The team can use data in **Table 1** to assist with setting short-terms goals and would delve into the literature for more comprehensive comparative data tables once their final choices were made.

SUMMARY

To evaluate the impact of evidence-based practice and understand the implications for your clinical decisions, a structured approach to measuring outcomes is essential. There are a number of valid (and highly reliable) instruments that can provide information on pain and disability in hand surgery and therapy practice. These measures should augment but not replace traditional physical impairment measures. The plan for measuring outcomes developed for your specific clinical practice must be customized to address your needs, taking into account staff support and the intended use of the information.

REFERENCES

1. Barbier O, Penta M, Thonnard JL. Outcome evaluation of the hand and wrist according to the international classification of functioning, disability, and health. Hand Clin 2003;19(3):371–8, vii.

2. Cieza A, Geyh S, Chatterji S, et al. ICF linking rules: an update based on lessons learned. J Rehabil Med 2005;37(4):212–8.

3. Cieza A, Brockow T, Ewert T, et al. Linking health-status measurements to the international classification of functioning, disability and health. J Rehabil Med 2002;34(5):205–10.

4. Cieza A, Stucki G. New approaches to understanding the impact of musculoskeletal conditions. Best Pract Res Clin Rheumatol 2004;18(2):141–54.

5. Cieza A, Stucki G. Understanding functioning, disability, and health in rheumatoid arthritis: the

basis for rehabilitation care. Curr Opin Rheumatol 2005;17(2):183–9.

6. Coenen M, Cieza A, Stamm TA, et al. Validation of the international classification of functioning, disability and health (ICF) core set for rheumatoid arthritis from the patient perspective using focus groups. Arthritis Res Ther 2006;8(4):R84.

7. Harris JE, MacDermid JC, Roth J. The International Classification of Functioning as an explanatory model of health after distal radius fracture: a cohort study. Health Qual Life Outcomes 2005;3(1):73.

8. Available at: http://www3.who.int/icf/icftemplate.cfm?myurl=homepage.html&mytitle=Home%20Page. International Classification of Functioning, Disability and Health. Available at: http://www3.who.int/icf/icftemplate.cfm?myurl=homepage.html&mytitle=Home%20Page. 2003. World Health Organization. 10-30-2006.

9. Michlovitz SL, LaStayo PC, Alzner S, et al. Distal radius fractures: therapy practice patterns. J Hand Ther 2001;14(4):249–57.

10. Law M, MacDermid JC. Evidence-based rehabilitation: a guide to practice. 2nd edition. Philadelphia: Slack Publishing; 2008.

11. Bellamy N, Campbell J, Haraoui B, et al. Clinimetric properties of the AUSCAN Osteoarthritis Hand Index: an evaluation of reliability, validity and responsiveness. Osteoarthr Cartil 2002;10(11):863–9.

12. MacDermid JC, Drosdowech D, Faber K. Responsiveness of self-report scales in patients recovering from rotator cuff surgery. J Shoulder Elbow Surg 2006;15(4):407–14.

13. Hunsaker FG, Cioffi DA, Amadio PC, et al. The American Academy of Orthopaedic Surgeons outcomes instruments: normative values from the general population. J Bone Joint Surg Am 2002;84-A(2):208–15.

14. American Academy of Orthopaedic Surgeons. American Academy of Orthopaedic Surgery. Available at: www.aaos.org/research/normstdy/main.cfm. 2003.

15. Solway S, Beaton DE, McConnell S, et al. The DASH outcome measure user's manual. 2nd edition. Toronto: Institute for Work and Health; 2002.

16. Beaton DE, Bombardier C, Katz JN, et al. Looking for important change/differences in studies of responsiveness. OMERACT MCID working group. Outcome measures in rheumatology. Minimal clinically important difference. J Rheumatol 2001;28(2):400–5.

17. Beaton DE, Boers M, Wells GA. Many faces of the minimal clinically important difference (MCID): a literature review and directions for future research. Curr Opin Rheumatol 2002;14(2):109–14.

18. Guyatt G, Walter S, Norman G. Measuring change over time: assessing the usefulness of evaluative instruments. J Chronic Dis 1987;40(2):171–8.

19. Jaeschke R, Singer J, Guyatt GH. Measurement of health status: ascertaining the minimal clinically important difference. Control Clin Trials 1989;10:407–15.

20. Brozek JL, Guyatt GH, Schunemann HJ. How a well-grounded minimal important difference can enhance transparency of labelling claims and improve interpretation of a patient reported outcome measure. Health Qual Life Outcomes 2006;4:69.

21. Guyatt G, Feeny D, Patrick D. Issues in quality-of-life measurement in clinical trials. Control Clin Trials 1991;12:81S–90S.

22. Norman GR, Sridhar FG, Guyatt GH, et al. Relation of distribution- and anchor-based approaches in interpretation of changes in health-related quality of life. Med Care 2001;39(10):1039–47.

23. Ozyurekoglu T, McCabe SJ, Goldsmith LJ, et al. The minimal clinically important difference of the Carpal Tunnel Syndrome symptom severity scale. J Hand Surg [Am] 2006;31(5):733–8.

24. Salaffi F, Stancati A, Silvestri CA, et al. Minimal clinically important changes in chronic musculoskeletal pain intensity measured on a numerical rating scale. Eur J Pain 2004;8(4):283–91.

25. Wells G, Anderson J, Beaton D, et al. Minimal clinically important difference module: summary, recommendations, and research agenda. J Rheumatol 2001;28(2):452–4.

26. Beaton DE, Katz JN, Fossel AH, et al. Measuring the whole or the parts? validity, reliability, and responsiveness of the disabilities of the arm, shoulder and hand outcome measure in different regions of the upper extremity. J Hand Ther 2001;14(2):128–46.

27. MacDermid JC, Roth JH, McMurtry R. Predictors of time lost from work following a distal radius fracture. J Occup Rehabilr 2007;17(1):47–62.

28. MacDermid JC, Solomon P, Law M, et al. Defining the effect and mediators of two knowledge translation strategies designed to alter knowledge, intent and clinical utilization of rehabilitation outcome measures: a study protocol. Implement Sci 2006;1(1):14 [NCT00298727].

29. MacDermid JC, Wessel J, Humphrey R, et al. Validity of self-report measures of pain and disability for persons who have undergone arthroplasty for osteoarthritis of the carpometacarpal joint of the hand. Osteoarthr Cartil 2007;15(5):524–30.

30. Massy-Westropp N, Krishnan J, Ahern M. Comparing the AUSCAN osteoarthritis hand index, Michigan hand outcomes questionnaire, and sequential occupational dexterity assessment for patients with rheumatoid arthritis. J Rheumatol 2004;31(10):1996–2001.

31. Kjeken I, Slatkowsky-Christensen B, Kvien TK, et al. Norwegian version of the Canadian occupational performance measure in patients with hand

osteoarthritis: validity, responsiveness, and feasibility. Arthritis Rheum 2004;51(5):709–15.

32. Kjeken I, Dagfinrud H, Slatkowsky-Christensen B, et al. Activity limitations and participation restrictions in women with hand osteoarthritis: patients descriptions, and associations between dimensions of functioning. Ann Rheum Dis 2005;64(11):1633–8.

33. Schmitt JS, Di Fabio RP. Reliable change and minimum important difference (MID) proportions facilitated group responsiveness comparisons using individual threshold criteria. J Clin Epidemiol 2004; 57(10):1008–18.

34. Apard T, Saint-Cast Y [Results of a 5 years follow-up of Arpe prosthesis for the basal thumb osteoarthritis]. Chir Main 2007;26(2):88–94.

35. Citron N, Hulme CE, Wardle N. A self-administered questionnaire for basal osteoarthritis of the thumb. J Hand Surg Eur Vol 2007;32(5):524–8.

36. Olivier LC, Gensigk F, Board TN, et al. Arthrodesis of the distal interphalangeal joint: description of a new technique and clinical follow-up at 2 years. Arch Orthop Trauma Surg 2008;128(3):307–11.

37. De Smet L, Robijns F, Degreef I. Outcome of proximal row carpectomy. Scand J Plast Reconstr Surg Hand Surg 2006;40(5):302–6.

38. Rothe M, Rudolf KD, Partecke BD [Long-term results following denervation of the wrist in patients with stages II and III SLAC-/SNAC-wrist]. Handchir Mikrochir Plast Chir 2006;38(4):261–6.

39. Naidu SH, Poole J, Horne A. Entire flexor carpi radialis tendon harvest for thumb carpometacarpal arthroplasty alters wrist kinetics. J Hand Surg [Am] 2006;31(7):1171–5.

40. Pegoli L, Zorli IP, Pivato G, et al. Scaphotrapeziotrapezoid joint arthritis: a pilot study of treatment with the scaphoid trapezium pyrocarbon implant. J Hand Surg [Br] 2006;31(5):569–73.

41. Rab M, Gohritz A, Gohla T, et al [Long-term results after resection arthroplasty in patients with arthrosis of the thumb carpometacarpal joint: comparison of abductor pollicis longus and flexor carpi radialis tendon suspension]. Handchir Mikrochir Plast Chir 2006;38(2):98–103.

42. De Smet L, Vaes F, Van Den BJ. Arthrodesis of the trapeziometacarpal joint for basal joint osteoarthritis of the thumb: the importance of obtaining osseous union. Chir Main 2005;24(5):222–4.

43. De Smet L, Sioen W, Spaepen D, et al. Total joint arthroplasty for osteoarthritis of the thumb basal joint. Acta Orthop Belg 2004;70(1):19–24.

44. Van Giffen N, Van Ransbeeck H, De Smet L. Stabilization of the pre-arthritic trapeziometacarpal joint using ligament reconstruction. Chir Main 2002; 21(5):277–81.

45. Angst F, John M, Goldhahn J, et al. Comprehensive assessment of clinical outcome and quality of life after resection interposition arthroplasty of the thumb saddle joint. Arthritis Rheum 2005;53(2): 205–13.

46. Jones G, Cooley HM, Bellamy N. A cross-sectional study of the association between Heberden's nodes, radiographic osteoarthritis of the hands, grip strength, disability and pain. Osteoarthr Cartil 2001;9(7):606–11.

47. Allen KD, DeVellis RF, Renner JB, et al. Validity and factor structure of the AUSCAN Osteoarthritis Hand Index in a community-based sample. Osteoarthr Cartil 2007;15(7):830–6.

48. MacDermid JC, Tottenham V. Responsiveness of the disability of the arm, shoulder, and hand (DASH) and patient-rated wrist/hand evaluation (PRWHE) in evaluating change after hand therapy. J Hand Ther 2004;17(1):18–23.

49. Atroshi I, Gummesson C, Andersson B, et al. The Disabilities of the Arm, Shoulder and Hand (DASH) outcome questionnaire: reliability and validity of the Swedish version evaluated in 176 patients. Acta Orthop Scand 2000;71(6):613–8.

50. Mathiowetz V, Kashman N, Volland G, et al. Grip and pinch strength: normative data for adults. Arch Phys Med Rehabil 1985;66:69–74.

51. MacDermid JC, Alyafi T, Richards RS, et al. Test-retest reliability of isometric strength and endurance grip tests performed on the Jamar and NK devices. Physiother Can 2003;53(1):48–54.

52. MacDermid JC, Mule M. Concurrent validity of the NK hand dexterity test. Physiother Res Int 2001; 6(2):83–93.

53. MacDermid JC, Evenhuis W, Louzon M. Inter-instrument reliability of pinch strength scores. J Hand Ther 2001;14(1):36–42.

54. Lang CE, Edwards DF, Birkenmeier RL, et al. Estimating minimal clinically important differences of upper-extremity measures early after stroke. Arch Phys Med Rehabil 2008;89(9):1693–700.

55. MacDermid JC, Roth JH, Rampersaud YR, et al. Trapezial arthroplasty with silicone rubber implantation for advanced osteoarthritis of the trapeziometacarpal joint of the thumb. Can J Surg 2003;46(2): 103–10.

The Use of Economic Evaluation in Hand Surgery

Achilleas Thoma, MD, MSc, FRCSC, FACS[a,b,c,*],
Leslie McKnight, MSc[d], Casey Knight, MD[e]

KEYWORDS

- Cost-effectiveness analysis • Cost-utility analysis
- Economic evaluation • Economic analysis
- Scaphoid fracture

Hand surgeons are constantly inundated with new techniques or approaches to solving hand problems. The average surgeon often faces difficulty in deciding when to adopt these new innovations, which may have been introduced at a recent conference or in the latest edition of a hand journal. Their decisions are more problematic when conflicting opinions are presented by experts. Whether working in the community or at an academic center, hand surgeons who are considering the adoption of a new approach to solving a particular hand problem (and abandoning a prevailing approach) need to consider the opportunity cost. Opportunity cost is defined as "the value of the forgone benefits" because the resource is not available for its best alternative use. It is, therefore, important that the hand surgeon, in addition to considering the risks and benefits of a procedure, weigh the benefits provided by the introduction of the new technology. Is it worth spending the limited resources available to their hospital or organization? The hand surgeons of today are expected to adopt evidence-based surgery principles in their practices.[1] It is expected that hand surgeons today behave as a manager of the health care system under they work. Being "manager" is one of the seven "Can Meds" competencies the Royal College of Physicians and Surgeons of Canada mandated of all residency training programs.[2]

Hand surgeons can use an economic analysis to determine if the new technique they would like to adopt is a cost-effective option. Economic analysis is a set of formal, quantitative methods used to compare alternative strategies with respect to their resource use and their expected outcomes.[3] There are four commonly quoted types of economic evaluations in the literature: 1) cost analysis (CA) (cost comparison study; not a full economic evaluation); 2) cost-effectiveness analysis (CEA); 3) cost-utility analysis (CUA); 4) cost-benefit analysis (CBA).[3,4]

In the initial design phase of an economic evaluation, the eventual type of analysis (CA, CEA, CUA) may not been known unless the effectiveness (ie, outcome) of both treatments has already been established in the literature. For instance, if the clinical outcomes of two competing techniques in digital replantation are the same (ie, successful replantations with similar probabilities of success and failures), then the study will be simplified to a CA or cost-comparison study. In this situation,

[a] Division of Plastic Surgery, Department of Surgery, McMaster University, St. Joseph's Healthcare, 304-43 Charlton Avenue East, Hamilton, Ontario L8N 1Y3, Canada
[b] Department of Clinical Epidemiology and Biostatistics, McMaster University, Biostatistics Unit/FSORC, St. Joseph's Healthcare, 50 Charlton Avenue East, Hamilton, Ontario L8N 4A6, Canada
[c] Surgical Outcomes Research Center (SOURCE), McMaster University, St. Joseph's Healthcare, 50 Charlton Avenue East, Hamilton, Ontario L8N 4A6, Canada
[d] Department of Surgery, Division of Plastic and Reconstructive Surgery, McMaster University, St. Joseph's Healthcare, 304-43 Charlton Avenue East, Hamilton, Ontario L8N 1Y3, Canada
[e] Division of Plastic and Reconstructive Surgery, Department of Surgery, McMaster University, St. Joseph's Healthcare, Hamilton, Ontario, Canada
* Corresponding author. 101-206 James Street S, Hamilton, ON L8P 3A9 Canada.
E-mail address: athoma@mcmaster.ca (A. Thoma).

Hand Clin 25 (2009) 113–123
doi:10.1016/j.hcl.2008.10.001

hand.theclinics.com

the less costly, yet equally effective, treatment option should be considered.[4]

If differences in effectiveness between the two techniques are identified in the course of the study, then the study can be designated as a CEA, CUA or CBA depending on how the consequences (outcomes) were measured (see **Table 1** for the main differences). If natural units were used (ie, successful replants, successful flaps, hospitalization days, and days to return to work), then the economic analysis would be labeled as CEA. If the outcomes were measured as quality adjusted life years (QALYs), the study would be labeled as CUA. If the outcomes were measured in dollars or pounds, then the study would be labeled as CBA.[3,4]

Economic evaluations can be divided into two methodological types. The first type, called a deterministic analysis, is one in which primary data are lacking and modeling is used. Data are obtained indirectly from the literature, usually by pooling the published evidence. From these data, researchers estimate the expected costs and expected benefits of the interventions by multiplying the costs and consequences by their probability of occurrence. The second type of evaluation, and most accurate one, is one in which researchers have primary data with means and standard deviations. This type is called a stochastic analysis. In a stochastic analysis, primary outcome data in both costs and consequences is obtained directly from patients.[1,4] Unfortunately, this type of analysis is seldom performed in hand surgery, probably because of the extra effort and time required to perform it. Hopefully, in the future this type of analysis will prevail.[4]

This article assists users of clinical research to search for and, in particular, appraise articles in the hand surgery literature that are purported to include a cost-effectiveness analysis. In addition, clinical researchers can learn to undertake cost-effectiveness analysis in hand surgery themselves.

Table 1
Distinguishing characteristics of the four main economic evaluations (cost-analysis, cost-effectiveness analysis, cost-utility analysis, and cost-benefit analysis)

Type of Analysis	Valuation of Costs	Identification of Outcomes (Consequences)	Metric Used in the Analysis
Cost-analysis	Monetary units (ie, $, £)	None	None. This analysis is only a comparison of costs
Cost-effectiveness analysis (CEA)	Monetary units (ie, $,£)	Common effect of interest. Common outcomes to the competing surgical interventions but with different degree of success (ie, successful flaps, successful replants, lives saved, sick days averted, hospital days averted)	$ per natural unit (ie, $ per successful replant, $ per life saved, $ per hospital day averted)
Cost-utility analysis (CUA)	Monetary units (ie, $, £)	Single or multiple effects that are not necessarily common to both interventions. Outcomes are measured in utilities that are transformed to Quality Adjusted Life Years (QALYs)	$ per QALY or £ per QALY
Cost-benefit analysis (CBA)	Monetary units (ie, $, £)	Single or multiple effects not necessarily common to both surgical procedures and are calculated in $ or £	Monetary units (ie, $ or £)

From Thoma A, Strumas N, Rockwell G, McKnight L. The use of cost-effectiveness analysis in plastic surgery clinical research. Clin Plast Surg 2008;35(2):285–96; with permission.

CLINICAL SCENARIO

A 40-year-old accountant is referred to a hand surgeon with an undisplaced fracture of the waist of his right scaphoid carpal bone. The injury happened on the weekend when the patient fell on his outstretched hand while playing baseball with some friends. Clinically, he has tenderness over the anatomic snuffbox and the radiographs reveal an undisplaced fracture. Based on the radiograph and clinical findings, the hand surgeon recommends an above elbow cast immobilization for 8 weeks, followed by another 4 weeks of below elbow casting. The patient, however, questions this treatment as his friend suffered exactly the same injury to his scaphoid one year ago also playing baseball, yet he underwent surgery "with a pin placed in his bone." The patient wonders why the recommendation to him is different. The surgeon tells him that surgery is unnecessary because the results are the same and, furthermore, surgery is a lot more expensive for him and the health care system. While revealing this to the patient, the surgeon recalls the words of a visiting professor at last month's academic rounds who claimed that there is no evidence that most of the new innovations in hand surgery are cost-effective as compared with the old techniques. On the way home, the surgeon decides to check if there is any evidence that the open reduction and fixation (ORIF) of the scaphoid is more cost-effective than just cast immobilization.

THE SEARCH

The ideal article addressing the effectiveness of ORIF would be one that compares ORIF of the scaphoid with casting alone. In such a comparative study, the costs and outcomes (consequences) would have been valued and the study design would have been of high level evidence (ie, systematic review, preferably a meta-analysis of randomized controlled trials [RCTs]). Because such analyses are rare in the hand surgery literature, to determine the cost-effectiveness of the ORIF, one should identify any economic evaluation (preferably a RCT) that deals with this subject.[1] The peer-reviewed electronic database, Cochrane Library, is the best source of high quality articles that deal with both effectiveness and cost-effectiveness of novel interventions. In the Cochrane search window, one should set the limits to "title, abstract, and keywords" and enter the search terms "open reduction and fixation" and "scaphoid." One should further refine the search by prompting the search engine to only look for articles within the "NHS Economic Evaluation Database." The results of this search yield one article: "A cost/utility analysis of open reduction and internal fixation versus cast immobilization for acute nondisplaced mid-waist scaphoid fractures" by Davis and colleagues.[5] This is exactly the article needed.

APPRAISING THE ARTICLE

Now that a relevant article has been found, the task is to appraise the article and determine if the results are valid; if the costs and outcomes were appropriately measured; and finally, if the results are relevant to the clinician's practice? In teaching evidence-based surgery, the authors have used the approach to reviewing economic evaluations in surgery found in **Box 1**.[1]

ARE THE RESULTS VALID?
Did the Analysis Provide a Full Economic Comparison of Health Care Strategies?

When comparing a novel to a prevailing hand surgical intervention or strategy, a full economic evaluation should consider both the costs and the outcomes of both interventions. Frequently, the term "cost-effective" is used in the hand literature in an inappropriate way. Investigators perform a cost comparison of the competing interventions. If the investigators found that the new intervention is less costly, they recommend its adoption. However, this is only a partial economic analysis because it does not take into consideration the consequences (ie, outcomes) of the competing interventions, which may vary in terms of probability of success or failure and complications.

There are nine possible outcomes based on incremental cost and effectiveness of a given procedure over another (**Fig. 1**).[1,4] Some decisions are clear-cut. For instance, cell 1 of **Fig. 1** represents the case where the novel procedure is both less costly and more effective than the traditional technique, a win-win situation. In this situation, the novel technique should be adopted. Similarly, if a procedure falls into cell 2, where it is more expensive and less effective, it should be rejected. Many decisions, however, are not as straightforward. Most new surgical procedures fall into cell 7; they are more effective, but also more expensive.

Another way to illustrate the concept of cost-effectiveness is with the cost-effectiveness plane (**Fig. 2**).[6] Effectiveness is shown on the horizontal axis and cost along the vertical axis. If the new surgical intervention falls in the right lower quadrant, there is a win-win scenario because the new intervention is both less expensive and more effective. If it falls in the left upper quadrant, it is rejected because it costs more and it is less effective, a lose-lose scenario. Most new procedures fall in the right upper quadrant (ie, more costly and more effective).[6]

The article by Davis and colleagues was a deterministic CUA. Costs of treatment by provider and facilities as well as productivity costs were calculated. The outcomes were measured in utilities and transformed into QALYs using the following formula:

$$QALY = (duration\ of\ health\ state)$$
$$\times\ (utility\ of\ health\ state)$$
$$+\ (future\ remaining\ life\ expectancy$$
$$-\ duration\ of\ health\ state)$$
$$\times\ (utility\ of\ successful\ reconstruction)$$

The QALY integrates changes in quantity of life (ie, reduction of mortality) and quality of life (ie, reduction in morbidity) into a standard "metric." Because both costs and consequences were measured, this study is considered a full economic evaluation.

Were All Relevant Viewpoints Considered?

When conducting an economic evaluation in hand surgery, researchers need to state explicitly who is benefiting from the adoption of the novel hand intervention or strategy. Is it the patient, the surgeon, the hospital, some third party payer or the society? The benefits obtained from a hand surgery intervention are not the same across all possible beneficiaries. For example, with the use of endoscopic carpal tunnel release (ECTR) for carpal tunnel release over the open carpal tunnel release technique, the hospital may be taking a loss because ECTR consumes greater resources. Conversely, a surgeon may benefit from higher remuneration using the ECTR technique. The patient runs a higher risk for neuropraxia of the median nerve with the ECTR and, hence, this procedure may not confer any advantage to the patient.[6] Ideally, one should consider all the relevant perspectives. For those who are concerned with the allocation of scarce health care resources, the most important perspective is that of the society and investigators should try to include this perspective in their analysis.

Davis and colleagues claimed to have taken a societal perspective. Costs were calculated using Medicare data and the Medicare resource-based relative value scale which assigns relative value units to various medical interventions based on current procedural termininology codes.[7,8] Surgeon and anesthesiologist fees were added to the hospital costs. The patient's cost of lost wages was estimated using average wages from the U.S. Bureau of Labor Statistics. On the surface, the costs measured seem to satisfy the consideration of the societal perspective. However, on careful review of their article and, in particular, the section on lost productivity on page 1228, there is concern that they did not meet all the criteria of a societal perspective because not all indirect costs have been accounted for. In addition to the productivity losses, a patient with an ORIF of the scaphoid is expected to have more pain

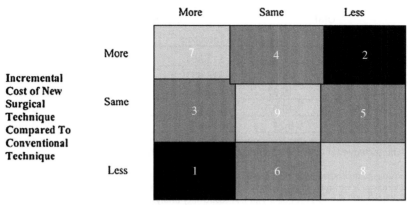

Fig. 1. Nine possible outcomes when comparing the new surgical technique and the conventional surgical technique. (*From* Thoma A, Sprague S, Tandan V. Users guide to the surgical literature: how to use an article on economic analysis. Can J Surg 2001;44:347; with permission.)

than a patient with cast immobilization. The cost of pain medication needs to be considered in the analysis, as well as other various personal expenses such as transportation, personal care or childcare, which may be different in the two treatments. Patients who have cast immobilization may go home by taxi or public transportation from the clinic. In the case of ORIF, the patient's spouse may have to take time off work to drive the patient to and from the hospital after a general anesthetic. Ideally, these indirect costs should be considered in an economic evaluation. Understandably, Davis and colleagues could not realistically capture all the indirect costs because their analysis was deterministic. To capture all the indirect costs, one has to

perform a prospective study and collect costs parallel to the trial.[1,4]

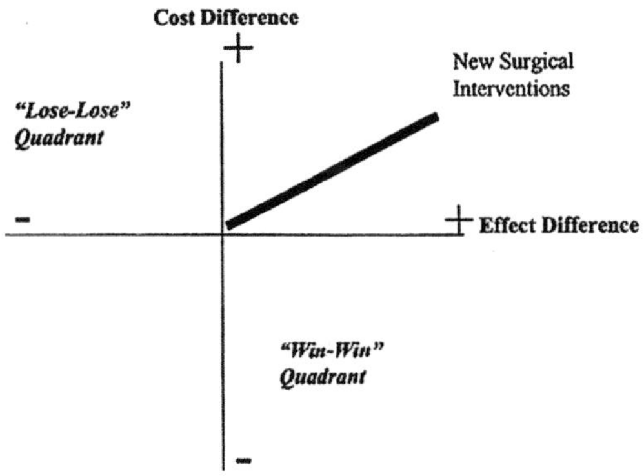

Were All the Relevant Clinical Strategies Compared?

It is important that an economic analysis considers the relevant strategies in the comparison of the two competing hand surgery interventions. The fact that patients may have a different baseline risk should be included in the analysis. To assess baseline risk, investigators should have reviewed all the previously published primary data comparing the two interventions. Preferably a systematic review or meta-analysis (if possible) should have been conducted to pool the primary data.

Fractures of the scaphoid and subsequent treatment may carry different risk factors for different population of patients. Davis and colleagues, to their credit, did such an analysis. They calculated the costs and outcomes (utilities) for four different age groups (**Table 2**). Although Davis and colleagues mentioned that: "scaphoid fractures account for 70 percent of all carpal fractures occurring most commonly in young men of working age," they did not consider worker's compensation board (WCB) cases in their analysis. It could be that the costs associated with WCB may be much different from Medicare and the conclusion of the economic analysis may be much different. This information would have been useful for hand surgeons and third party payers. This point is a weakness in this study. Additionally, the ORIF of the scaphoid can be achieved by various techniques (ie, single K-wire, parallel K-wires, regular cancellous screws, or Herbert screws). The article by Davis was not explicit as to the technique used.

Fig. 2. Cost effectiveness plane. (*From* Thoma A, Haines T, Veltri K, et al. A methodological guide to performing a cost-utility study comparing surgical techniques. Can J Plast Surg 2004;12:179–87; with permission.)

Table 2
Comparison of total cost, utilities, and incremental cost/utility ratios across age groups

| Age | ORIF | | Casting | | |
	Total cost[a]	QALYs	Total cost[a]	QALYs	IGUR: ORIF versus casting
25 years	$7940	25.89	$13,851	25.68	ORIF dominates[b]
35 years	$7940	23.27	$13,851	23.09	ORIF dominates
45 years	$7940	19.77	$13,851	19.63	ORIF dominates
55 years	$7940	15.07	$13,851	14.97	ORIF dominates
65 years	$7942	8.74	$13,651	8.70	ORIF dominates

Abbreviations: ICIR, incremental cost/utility radio; ORIF, open reduction and internal fixation; QALYs, quality-adjusted life-years.
  [a] Total cost includes lost productivity and direct medical costs.
  [b] A dominant strategy is defined as one that is less costly and more effective.
  From Davis EN, Chung KC, Kotsis SV, et al, S Vijan. A cost/utility analysis of open reduction and internal fixation versus cast immobilization for acute nondisplaced mid-waist scaphoid fractures. Plast Reconstr Surg 2006;117:1223–35; with permission.

WERE THE COSTS AND OUTCOMES PROPERLY MEASURED AND VALUED?
Was Clinical Effectiveness Established?

The ideal study to show the effectiveness of the competing hand interventions would be a meta-analysis of multiple RCTs.[9] If a meta-analysis is not available, then one should look for individual RCTs that compare the effectiveness of the interventions if such exist. An RCT will have high internal validity but may not be generalizable if the inclusion criteria were too restrictive. Unfortunately, meta-analyses and RCTs are not common in the hand surgery literature. In this situation, one can pool data from lower level evidence study designs such as prospective cohort or case series. Another approach to this dilemma is the use of modeling. Modeling studies can make projections of long-term outcomes from short-term trial data relating to intermediate end points that can be used to offset this problem of inadequate follow-up. The Markov model is such an example, but discussion of this is beyond the scope of this article.[3]

In the study by Davis and colleagues, the effectiveness was measured by obtaining utilities (ie, preferences) of the various health states associated with scaphoid fractures (ie, successful union, nonunion with repeat surgery). They used the "time trade-off" (TTO) technique to obtain utilities (preferences) associated with the health states of the two competing strategies (ORIF versus cast immobilization).

With the TTO, participants are presented with the hypothetical scenarios. For example, choice A is associated with a shortened life expectancy of x years due to complications after surgery and choice B, with a given life expectancy of t years.

In other words, patients are asked about how much of their life expectancy they would be willing to trade-off to avoid the health state denoted by choice B. The utility value of the health state in question is estimated by the proportion between the shortened life expectancy x and the full life expectancy of the intermediate outcome t.[10]

To assess patient preferences, Davis and colleagues randomly selected 50 University of Michigan medical students to complete an Internet-based TTO questionnaire. Ideally, they should have used their TTO questionnaire with the general public or with patients who experienced scaphoid fractures in the past. One may be suspicious that the University of Michigan medical students' preferences may not reflect those of the general public or the patients with scaphoid fractures. The authors acknowledged this limitation. Obtaining utilities from the general public would have been difficult. Explanation of the various health states associated with the scaphoid fractures and treatment to the general public is an arduous task. Davis and colleagues transformed the utilities into QALYs, which is the acceptable metric for performing a CUA.

Were the Costs Measured Accurately?

The measurement of the costs of the two competing hand interventions will depend on the perspective taken in the analysis. For example, if one takes the hospital's perspective, the patient's productivity losses are not relevant. In other words, the hospital won't be concerned if a patient has to pay somebody to care for them once they leave the hospital. The hospital is only concerned with the costs incurred while there and receiving treatment. When the costs are reported, it is important that they be reported in the physical quantities or resources consumed separately from the prices. The reason is that the price per quantity of resource consumed is different in many jurisdictions (ie, states, provinces and countries). By this method of reporting, health economists and hand surgeons in other jurisdictions can make their own calculations and decide for themselves if a novel intervention is cost-effective or not in their geographic area. Another problem that complicates an analysis is the publication of charges of a particular intervention, which may be different from the actual costs. For example, what a patient pays to a hospital for ECTR is usually higher than the actual cost to perform the surgery. This discrepancy is more problematic in the United States where many hospitals work on a profit business model as compared with the Canadian socialized health care system where there is only one third party payer (the government). In a recent study, Taira and colleagues[11] compared four methods of estimating costs in three separate trials involving percutaneous coronary revascularization They included: 1) hospital charges; 2) hospital charges converted to costs by use of hospital-level cost–to-charge ratios; 3) hospital charges converted to costs by use of department-level cost-to-charge ratios; and 4) itemized laboratory costs with non-procedural hospital costs generated from department-level cost-to-charge ratios. The authors found that although there were big differences in the magnitude of the estimates obtained by the various methods, the method used to approximate costs did not affect the main results of the economic comparisons of any of the trials. They also concluded that conversion of hospital charges to costs on the basis of department-level cost-to-charge ratios appears to represent a reasonable compromise between accuracy and ease of implementation.[4,11]

When reporting the results of an economic evaluation, it is important that the clinical investigators tabulate the quantity of the resources used in their natural units instead of summarizing the costs (eg, operating room time in hours, hospital days, days to return to work, etc). By adding the natural units, future investigators in other states, provinces, or countries can take the resource use from this study and "plug in" their costs/unit of resources in their setting. In this way, they can decide if the novel hand technique is cost-effective or not.

Davis and colleagues estimated the medical costs by using the Medicare resource-based relative value scale which assigns relative value units to various medical interventions based on current procedural terminology codes.[7,8] They used the fee schedule for the 2003 calendar year and the

geographic practice cost index for Michigan locality 01 to calculate the Medicare physician payment. For anesthesia services, they used a separate formula that was also geographically adjusted; it was based on the time required to manage each ORIF of the scaphoid and to deal with the complications (health states) associated with the procedure. To these, they added the hospital costs based on Medicare payments. Finally, they added the lost productivity costs. Overall, the methodology chosen to calculate the costs is satisfactory. They also provided the probabilities of the "health states" associated with management of the scaphoid fracture (see **Table 1**). These probabilities are not confirmed as accurate, however. Ideally, the identification of the probabilities should come from a systematic review in which at least two independent reviewers examine the literature to ensure that no important articles relevant to this study were omitted. The time horizon under consideration needs to be explained as well. Did the study take into account short-, intermediate- or long-term outcome costs into consideration? The authors, to their credit, readily admitted that they "did not consider time off from work caused by arthritis, which is a late complication, because of the variable effect that arthritis has on a patient's ability to work." The issue of productivity losses is only partially correct because they did not account for all indirect costs except wage losses.

Were the Data on Costs and Outcomes Appropriately Integrated?

Many published studies in the surgical literature that purport to be CEA or CUA actually are not. The usual mistake is that investigators estimate the direct medical costs and compare them to each other. If the direct costs are less with the novel technique, then they proclaim that the novel technique is cost-effective. The second error is to take a ratio of cost and effect of the novel intervention and compare it to that of the comparative intervention. When a comparison is made between two competing interventions, one is interested in determining the extra benefit that is gained from the extra unit cost. This is obtained by calculating the incremental cost utility ratio (ICUR). The ICUR represents the marginal cost per marginal unit of utility and is calculated as follows:

$$ICUR = \Delta C / \Delta U = \text{Mean Cost}_{novel}$$
$$- \text{Mean Cost}_{comparative}) /$$
$$(\text{Mean QALY}_{novel}$$
$$- \text{Mean QALY}_{comparative}$$

This ratio, which integrates costs and effectiveness, tells us whether to adopt the novel procedure. The result is represented as cost per QALY. In simple words, it shows how much it costs to prolong the life of a patient by one extra year in perfect health. The higher the ICUR, the greater the incremental cost for an additional healthy year of life.[4] It is generally accepted that if an intervention has an ICUR below the threshold of $20,000/QALY, there is a strong indication for its acceptance. Alternatively, if the ICUR is above the threshold of $100,000/QALY, there is an indication for its rejection.[12] For ICURs falling in-between, the adoption will depend on the circumstances of the patient, surgeon, and center, as well as the affordability. For example, composite tissue transplantation of the hand may have an ICUR well above the threshold, but if it is performed infrequently, then it will be of no great consequence to the society. Conversely, hand transplantation costs at the societal level may be dwarfed by a procedure that is less expensive at the level of the individual case, such as an ECTR, which because of its frequency, cumulatively may cost more to society.[13]

When considering costs, the concept of discounting must be addressed. The costs and benefits of a surgical intervention or health care program may not occur at the same time point. The future costs and benefits need to be considered in an economic evaluation because costs in the future will not be the same as costs today. Discounting is the process of determining the present value of the costs and benefits as experienced in future. Discounting is based on a time preference that is shared; in this society, most people prefer to experience the benefits now and pay later (even if there were no interest rates or inflation). Therefore, discounting places a higher weighting on current costs and benefits than on those experienced in the uncertain future, and discounting is commonly quoted as 5% per annum.[3,4]

Davis and colleagues integrated the costs and consequences of the ORIF and casting of scaphoid fractures and provided us with an incremental cost-utility ratio (**Table 3**). The authors did not discuss the concept of discounting. It is assumed that their time horizon was one year, in which case discounting was not necessary.

Was Appropriate Allowance made for Uncertainties in the Analysis?

In an RCT comparing the outcomes of ORIF versus cast immobilization in the treatment of scaphoid fractures, each outcome measure would have a mean (average) effectiveness. If this RCT was coupled with an economic analysis, then the mean (average) cost of each outcome could be determined.[1,4] In such an ideal study design, one could calculate the ICUR of ORIF versus casting and determine if ORIF is cost-effective or not. Using the average QALY and average cost of each outcome to calculate the ICUR is not representative of the whole population as there is dispersion about the mean (ie, not all data points fall on the mean, some data points fall below or above the mean value). The standard deviation (SD) is a measurement of this dispersion (or spread) of data about the mean. In a sensitivity analysis, the

Table 3
Comparison of direct cost, utilities, and incremental cost/utility ratios results across age groups

Age	ORIF		Casting		IGUR[b]: ORIF versus casting
	Direct cost[a]	QALYs	Direct cost[a]	QALYs	
25 years	$1747	25.89	$605	25.68	$5438
35 years	$1747	23.27	$605	23.09	$6344
45 years	$1747	19.77	$605	19.63	$8157
55 years	$1747	15.07	$605	14.97	$11,420
65 years	$1599	8.74	$405	8.70	$29,850

Abbreviations: ICUR, incremental cost/utility radio; ORIF, open reduction and internal fixation; QALYs, quality-adjusted life-years.
[a] Direct excludes lost productivity and only includes direct medical costs (physician fees, anesthesia fees if applicable, and surgical center fees if applicable).
[b] ICUR = additional cost per QALY gained wish ORIF over casting.
From Davis EN, Chung KC, Kotsis SV, et al A cost/utility analysis of open reduction and internal fixation versus cast immobilization for acute nondisplaced mid-waist scaphoid fractures. Plast Reconstr Surg 2006;117:1223–35; with permission.

ICUR is recalculated using the best and worst case scenarios. For example, if the true costs are one SD above the mean, the ICUR is recalculated. One does the same for the effectiveness by considering the plausible scenario that the effectiveness is one SD below the mean. If, based on these assumptions, the ICUR is unchanged or remains below an acceptable threshold, then one can conclude the novel intervention is indeed cost-effective.

In a deterministic analysis such as the one in the Davis and colleagues article, the data are secondary and based on estimates that are imprecise. When uncertainty exists, a sensitivity analysis is required to assess the robustness of the results.[4] One would like to know the best case and the worse case scenario results based on some plausible assumptions about the probabilities of occurrence of the health states and costs under consideration. These corrections can be performed by adjusting the cost, utility, or probability of one variable at a time (one-way sensitivity analysis) or by varying multiple variables at the same time (two-way or multi-way analysis). If the final concluding results after the sensitivity analysis still fall within the same quadrant of the cost-effective plane (see **Fig. 1**) and below an acceptable threshold, then one can conclude that the results are considered robust and believable.[4]

Davis and associates—to their credit—did perform a sensitivity analysis to examine how robust their results are. A one-way sensitivity analysis to determine the effects of varying amounts of lost wages on the total cost of ORIF and casting was done. They performed a one-way sensitivity analysis to determine the effect of varying the utility for each health state on the difference in QALY between ORIF and casting. Another one-way sensitivity analysis was performed to examine the effects of varying the probabilities of each health state on total costs and QALYs. The authors found that changing the probability of the health state "arthritis" altered the QALYs of ORIF versus casting. This finding prompted the authors to conduct a two-way sensitivity analysis varying the probabilities of arthritis in ORIF and casting and the 25–64 year age group.

Are Estimates of Costs and Outcomes Related to the Baseline Risk in the Treatment Population?

The costs and outcomes of surgical procedures are related to the baseline risk of condition under study. For example, patients considered high risk may benefit more from a procedure than those individuals at low risk. Factors, such as age, may pose greater risk for certain conditions and therefore convey greater benefits for individuals receiving a particular procedure.

Davis and colleagues considered baseline risk by incorporating five different age group intervals (see **Table 3**). Their results revealed that younger patients experienced a relatively greater gain in QALY with ORIF.

WHAT ARE THE RESULTS?
What were the Incremental Costs and Outcomes of Each Strategy?

To determine the incremental costs and outcomes of each strategy, the tables in their article are viewed. **Table 2** compares the total costs, utilities, and ICURs across age groups. ORIF was more effective and less costly than casting in all age groups, with the greatest benefit observed in 25–34 years of age group (ORIF: QALY: 25.89; cost: $7940; versus casting: QALY: 25.68; cost: $13,851). ORIF dominated (less costly and more effective) as it fell in the right lower quadrant of the cost-effectiveness plane (see **Fig. 2**). These results were largely attributed to lost wages. The authors re-analyzed results using only direct costs (Medicare only) (see **Table 3**). In this analysis, ORIF was more effective, yet more costly, across all age groups than casting. The ORIF fell in the right upper quadrant of the cost-effectiveness plane. However, the ICUR was below the threshold of $20,000/QALY in all age groups except for patients who were older than 65 years of age.

Do Incremental Costs and Outcomes Differ Among Subgroups?

Looking at **Tables 2** and **3**, there are differences in incremental costs and outcomes among age subgroups. In **Table 2**, the QALYs decreased with increasing age for ORIF and casting. The total costs of ORIF and casting remained the same from 25–64 years of age and decreased slightly in the over 65 years of age group. In **Table 2**, the QALYs were unchanged from **Table 3** (QALYs decreased with increasing age). Total costs also remained the same from 25–64 years of age and decreased slightly in the over 65 years of age group. The ICUR of ORIF versus casting increased with increasing age from $5438 (25–34 years of age) to $29,850 (greater than 65 years of age).

How Much Does Allowance for Uncertainty Change the Results?

The results of the sensitivity analyses are found on pages 1231 and 1232 of the Davis article. **Table 3** describes the results of the one-way sensitivity analysis to determine the effects of lost wages on the total costs of ORIF and casting. The authors found that when a patient had greater than 16% of lost income, casting became more costly than ORIF, which was approximately 2.6 weeks with casting and 1.3 weeks with ORIF. Adjusting the utility of each health state did not have a significant effect on the difference in QALYs between ORIF and casting. Varying the probability of each health state did not affect the total direct costs of ORIF or casting. When varying the probability of the health state "arthritis" changes in QALY of ORIF versus casting were observed. A two-way sensitivity analysis was conducted to determine to effects of the varying the probabilities of arthritis in the different age groups (excluding the over 65 year group). The results of the two-way sensitivity analysis revealed that ORIF was more effective than casting in all age categories.

WILL THE RESULTS HELP ME IN CARING FOR MY PATIENTS?
Are the Treatment Benefits Worth the Harms and Costs?

Returning to **Fig. 2** (the cost-effectiveness plane), most novel procedures are more costly but more effective. In such cases, it is generally accepted that if an intervention has an ICUR below $20,000/QALY, there is a strong indication for its acceptance, whereas if the ICUR is above $100,000/QALY, there is an indication for its rejection.[12] There has been much discussion in the literature regarding the interpretation and application of the ICUR. In particular, the quantitative thresholds proposed by Laupacis and colleagues[12] in 1992 have been criticized for being arbitrary and out-dated, although they remain in frequent use.[14-16] For example, the National Institute for Health and Clinical Excellence (NICE) of the British National Health Service uses £20,000/QALY as their ICUR threshold for acceptance of new technologies.[17,18] There is an additional controversy regarding the $20,000/QALY threshold. As health care resources are scarce and as hand surgeons are working within a fixed budget, clinicians cannot implement all novel procedures whose ICUR is below $20,000/QALY. If they do, it will lead to an uncontrolled growth of health care spending. Some health economists believe that necessary conditions for implementing a new intervention are:[1] 1) it is truly a win-win situation (ie, it falls in the lower right quadrant of the cost-effectiveness plane);[2] 2) if it is more expensive yet more effective and less than $20,000/QALY, practitioners need to identify an existing intervention (hand procedure) or combinations of interventions (a number of hand procedures) to cancel or delete from our repertoire to generate the additional resources for the novel procedure.[19]

Davis and colleagues found the ICUR of ORIF versus casting to be lower than the threshold of $20,000/QALY in all age groups except in individuals over 65 years of age (ICUR $29,850/QALY). Therefore, ORIF is a cost-effective procedure compared with casting for individuals under the age of 65. The patient in the hypothetical scenario is 40 years of age, therefore, one expects him to benefit from ORIF.

Could a Clinician's Patients Expect Similar Health Outcomes?

To determine if a patient could expect similar results, clinicians need to ask two questions: 1) Is your treatment of acute scaphoid fractures similar to the treatments used in the study? 2) Are the patients in Davis and colleagues study similar to the patient being treated? Scaphoid fractures can be repaired with a number of techniques that include k-wires and Herbert screws. If a patient also receives the same ORIF technique as in the Davis and colleagues study, one would expect that the patient would benefit from this approach. The patient in the hypothetical scenario is a 40-year-old male. In the appraised article, the utilities, health state probabilities and costs were derived from different populations. The utilities were obtained from 50 medical students with a mean age of 23.7 years. A literature search was conducted to determine the health state probabilities. To determine the population used to derive the probabilities, the papers included in the review would need to be reviewed. The authors state that scaphoid fractures are most common in young adult male population and obtained the costs of loss wages for young adult men. There is no reason to believe that a patient is different from the population examined by Davis and colleagues, so it is assumed that a patient will also benefit from ORIF.

Could I Expect Similar Costs?

The cost of a surgical intervention is the summation of the resources used (eg, operating time, nursing staff time) and the unit price of each resource. The price per quantity of resource consumed is different in many jurisdictions (ie, states, provinces and countries). Davis and colleagues reported, in detail, the costs and utilities separately, allowing for surgeons in other jurisdictions to calculate their own ICUR. One can recalculate the ICUR based on the cost/quantity consumed applicable to our locale and if one finds, indeed, that it falls below $20,000/QALY, then one can prepare to accept ORIF as the strategy of choice.

RESOLUTION OF THE SCENARIO

Returning to the original scenario, we can proceed and advise our patient. We can tell the patient that the best evidence we have suggests that ORIF is a cost-effective strategy as compared with cast immobilization and this is what we recommend. We are cognizant, however, that this conclusion was based on a decision analytic model. The elusive truth is still out there, waiting for keen hand investigators to find it. The definitive truth to this question is a multi-center RCT comparing ORIF and cast immobilization piggy-backed to an economic evaluation. Parallel to the RCT, we collect both direct and indirect costs as a result of both strategies.[1,4]

REFERENCES

1. Thoma A, Sprague S, Tandan V. Users' guide to the surgical literature: how to use an article on economic analysis. Can J Surg 2001;44(5):347–54.
2. The Royal College of Physicians and Surgeons of Canada. The CanMeds assessment tools handbook: an introductory guide to assessment methods for the CanMEDS competencies. 1st edition. In: Bandiera G, Sherbino J, Frank JR, editors. Ottowa, Ontario (Canada): The Royal College of Physicians and Surgeons of Canada; 2006.
3. Drummond MF, Sculpher MJ, Torrance GW, et al. Methods for economic evaluation of health care programmes. 3rd edition. United Kingdom: Oxford University Press; 2005.
4. Thoma A, Strumas N, Rockwell G, et al. The use of cost-effectiveness analysis in plastic surgery clinical research. Clin Plast Surg 2008;35(2):285–96.
5. Davis EN, Chung KC, Kotsis SV, et al. A cost/utility analysis of open reduction and internal fixation versus cast immobilization for acute nondisplaced mid-waist scaphoid fractures. Plast Reconstr Surg 2006;117:1223–35.
6. Thoma A, Haines T, Veltri K, et al. A methodological guide to performing a cost-utility study comparing surgical techniques. Can J Plast Surg 2004;12:179–87.
7. American Medical Association. Current procedural terminology. Chicago: American Medical Association; 2003.
8. National physician fee schedule relative value units. Centers for Medicare and Medicaid Services. October 2003.
9. Sprague S, McKay P, Thoma A. Study designs and the hierarchy of evidence in clinical practice. Clin Plast Surg 2008;35(2):195–206.
10. Cugno S, Sprague S, Duku E, et al. Composite tissue allotransplantation of the face: decision analysis model. Can J Plast Surg 2007;15(3):145–52.
11. Taira DA, Seto TB, Seigrist R, et al. Comparison of analytic approaches for the economic evaluation of new technologies alongside multicenter clinical trials. Am Heart J 2003;145:452–8.
12. Laupacis A, Feeny D, Detsky AS, et al. How attractive does a technology have to be to warrant adoption and utilization? Tentative guidelines for using clinical and economic evaluations. Can Med Assoc J 1992;146:473–81.
13. Thoma A, McKnight L, McKay P, et al. Forming the research question. Clin Plast Surg 2008;35(2):189–94.
14. Asim O, Petrou S. Valuing a QALY: review of current controversies. Exp Rev Pharmacoeconomics Outcomes Res 2005;5:667–9.
15. McGregor M, Caro JJ. QALYs: are they helpful to decision makers? Pharmacoeconomics 2006;24:947–52.
16. Vijan S. Should we abandon QALYs as a resource allocation tool? Pharmacoeconomics 2006;24:953–4.
17. Pearson SD, Rawlins MD. Quality, innovation, and value for money: NICE and the British National Health Service. JAMA 2005;294:2618–22.
18. Buxton MJ. Economic evaluation and decision making in the UK. Pharmacoeconomics 2006;24:1133–42.
19. Gafni A, Birch S. Inclusion of drugs in provincial drug benefit programs: should "reasonable decisions" lead to uncontrolled growth in expenditures? CMAJ 2003;168(7):849–51.

Knowledge Translation: Putting the "Practice" in Evidence-Based Practice

Joy C. MacDermid, BScPT, PhD[a,b,*], Ian D. Graham, PhD[c,d]

KEYWORDS

- Knowledge translation • Implementation
- Practice change • Evidence-based practice
- Practice guidelines • Knowledge exchange

The fact that an opinion has been widely held is no evidence whatever that it is not utterly absurd; indeed in view of the silliness of the majority of mankind, a widespread belief is more likely to be foolish than sensible.
    —*Bertrand Russell, Marriage and Morals (1929), chapter 5; British author, mathematician, and philosopher (1872–1970)*
    Absence of evidence is not evidence of absence.
    —*Carl Sagan, American astronomer and popularizer of astronomy (1934–1996)*

Evidence-based hand surgery and therapy practice fall between the two pillars of dilemma exemplified above. Generalized opinions, or even our own uncontrolled clinical observations, can lead us to erroneous, even foolish, conclusions for many reasons. However, an overly rigid expectation that one can use high-quality evidence to make every clinical decision is equally foolhardy. In many instances, the ideal studies have not been conducted, and in many others, it may be practically impossible to do so. Therefore, clinicians must always act in an environment of uncertainty, using the best available evidence to support the process of an optimal clinical choice that integrates evidence from clinical research studies with the less tangible truths embedded in values, experiences, and expertise brought to the table by the clinician and the patient. Where this "balance" is not appreciated or reflected in actions taken, the process of evidence-based practice (EBP) is misappropriated and the outcomes are less likely to be satisfactory for all those involved.

EVIDENCE MUST BE MOVED INTO ACTION TO ACCOMPLISH HEALTH BENEFITS

You ask me why I do not write something.... I think one's feelings waste themselves in words, they ought all to be distilled into actions and into actions which bring results.
    —*Florence Nightingale, in Cecil Woodham-Smith, Florence Nightingale (1951); English nurse in Crimean War (1820–1910)*

EBP hinges on the assumption that once new (higher-quality) knowledge is generated, it will be applied/implemented. When knowledge is available and is not used, a gap is created between knowledge and practice or "action." Gaps between knowledge/evidence and actions in practice can exist for many reasons; some are justified,

Funded by a New Investigator Award, Canadian Institutes of Health Research.
[a] Hand and Upper Limb Centre Clinical Research Laboratory, St. Joseph's Health Centre, 268 Grosvenor Street, London, Ontario N6A 3A8, Canada
[b] School of Rehabilitation Science, LB33, McMaster University, Institute for Applied Health Sciences, Room 429, 1400 Main Street West, 4th Floor, Hamilton, Ontario L8S 1C7, Canada
[c] Knowledge Translation, Canadian Institutes of Health Research, 160 Elgin Street, Ottawa, Ontario K1A 0W9, Canada
[d] School of Nursing, University of Ottawa, Ontario K1H 8M5, Canada
* Corresponding author. Hand and Upper Limb Centre Clinical Research Laboratory, St. Joseph's Health Centre, 268 Grosvenor Street, London, Ontario N6A 3A8, Canada.
E-mail address: macderj@mcmaster.ca (J.C. MacDermid).

Hand Clin 25 (2009) 125–143
doi:10.1016/j.hcl.2008.10.003
0749-0712/08/$ – see front matter © 2009 Elsevier Inc. All rights reserved.

others are not. The need to determine whether this gap exists on an individual level is built into the EBP process, in which one compares his/her own clinical decisions with what best evidence suggests. But does a pervasive problem exist in hand surgery and therapy with evidence–practice gaps?

THE EVIDENCE–PRACTICE GAP IN HAND SURGERY AND THERAPY

The way to answer this question is to examine the evidence on practice patterns and compare them with the best available evidence. The authors looked for examples of where practice patterns had been studied and then compared those with the available evidence.

Perhaps the most studied aspect of practice attitudes and patterns is the use of hand surgery for the rheumatoid hand. Thanks to a series of surveys conducted by Alderman and Chung[1] and their co-investigators, we have some indication of the attitudes and practices of different end users of knowledge regarding hand surgery for the rheumatoid hand. In 2002, this group used administrative databases to assess surgical rates for fusion, joint replacement, and tenosynovectomy for patients coded as having a diagnosis of rheumatoid arthritis. Age/sex surgery rates by state were examined and revealed a 9- to 12-times variation across states in the use of the studied procedures. These variations were not explained by surgeon density. In addition, men were more likely to get early aggressive surgical interventions, whereas women were more likely to get end-stage reconstruction. Subsequently, the group looked at how patients felt about hand surgery and found that men and women were equally willing to have surgery and equally concerned about hand appearance, function, and pain.[2] Conversely, 73% of surgeons thought that women valued hand appearance more than did men. Another survey of hand surgeons and rheumatologists revealed that they disagreed significantly on the indications for these procedures.[3,4] More importantly, they disagreed significantly on the effectiveness of surgery. For example, 83% of hand surgeons, but only 34% of rheumatologists, believed that metacarpophalangeal (MCP) arthroplasty improves hand function.[3,4]

Next, the authors used clinical queries in PubMed to search "rheumatoid arthritis and hand surgery" (see the article on searching the evidence elsewhere in this issue) to locate randomized controlled trials on the effectiveness of hand surgery for the rheumatoid hand. The search provided 11 trials: 7 compared different MCP arthroplasty implant options to each other,[5–11] 1 evaluated the use of a supplemental surgical technique (crossed intrinsic transfer),[12] 1 evaluated the use of continuous passive motion[13] as an adjunct to hand therapy, and 2 were not relevant. Despite a tendency for underpowered and low-quality trials and a lack of difference between different treatment options, all studies suggested that hand function and pain are improved following MCP arthroplasty.

Therefore, a gap exists between the best available evidence and attitudes of physicians, in particular rheumatologists, about the effectiveness of MCP arthroplasty. A differential use of the intervention was indicated, suggesting a gap between evidence and behaviors (practice patterns). A gap was evident between patient-perceived needs and the perceptions of surgeons, which is reflected in differential delivery of services consistent with the surgeon bias. This scenario illustrates a substantial evidence–practice gap in one area of hand surgery practice and, thus, a need for different end users of information (patients, rheumatologists, and hand surgeons) to become more informed about the available evidence. Practice-based evidence is sufficient to suggest that all groups might potentially need to change their decision-making processes based on the current research evidence.

Perhaps rheumatoid arthritis is a unique problem, where transfer of knowledge is more complicated. Is this example representative? Although survey data on practice patterns are less available for other areas of practice, enough data exist to suggest a common trend. For example, although substantial work has been conducted on new flexor tendon suture techniques, a recent postal survey of all consultant plastic surgeons and consultant orthopedic surgeons who were members of the Irish Hand Surgery Society suggested that that the two-stranded Kessler core and simple running peripheral suture remains the most popular flexor tendon repair (for >70%).[14]

The trend in hand therapy is also similar. Despite considerable evidence that self-report outcome measures reflect important aspects of recovery and are more related to global outcome like return-to-work,[15] fewer than 10% of therapists reported using them.[16] The authors recently surveyed hand therapists on their practice patterns for tennis elbow and also conducted a systematic review of the literature[17] and found a considerable mismatch. Few studies support commonly used interventions like exercise and education, whereas high-quality evidence supports some rarely used techniques/modalities, (eg, Rebox).[17]

This evidence–practice gap is not unique to hand surgery/therapy. It exists across the health care system in the United States and other countries. It has been suggested that 30% to 45% of patients are not receiving care according to evidence and, of more concern, 20% to 50% of the care provided is not needed or potentially harmful,[18–20] differences that are not explained by sociodemographics.

This article deals with knowledge translation (KT), the link from evidence to action (practice). This new field builds on traditions, theories, and research from many different disciplines that have a common challenge to make things "work better" by ensuring that best approaches are implemented. For example, quality assurance, at least conceptually, deals with ensuring better practices are implemented within clinics. Engineers may discuss "technology transfer"; others call it "implementation science." Overall, more than 100 terms and definitions have been identified to describe this concept.

The authors use the following term and definition because it is comprehensive and drives the approaches they and their national health research funding agency use.

Knowledge translation is a dynamic and iterative process that includes synthesis, dissemination, exchange and ethically sound application of knowledge to improve the health of Canadians, provide more effective health services and products and strengthen the health care system.
  –Canadian Institutes of Health Research, available at: http://www.cihr-irsc.gc.ca/e/29,418.html.

The authors also like this brief definition: "Research use is the process by which specific research-based knowledge is implemented in practice."[21–23]

KNOWLEDGE-TO-ACTION CYCLE

KT is optimized if research informs practice and practice informs research, which is best accomplished by the engagement of knowledge developers and different end users in sustained partnerships that contribute to all aspects of the generation and use of new knowledge. This process has been well described in the knowledge-to-action (KTA) cycle (**Fig. 1**). It contains iterative cycles of knowledge creation and application (action). Knowledge creation can begin with individual research studies, be deepened through the synthesis of knowledge across different studies, and lead to tools that allow the knowledge to be applied or implemented. New knowledge is ready to be moved into action if evidence about "the right thing to do" is sufficient (not perfect). At the implementation stage, the focus is on making knowledge useable and more likely to be applied, which requires adapting the knowledge to the context, identifying and addressing local or system barriers to create changes in practice that can be sustained over time, and providing input into the next wave of knowledge generation. The success of this process must be monitored to assess whether both the behavior and the outcomes have changed. In fact, even within controlled trials, effects may be underestimated when little attention is directed toward assuring or measuring treatment fidelity.

WHY DO EVIDENCE–PRACTICE GAPS EXIST? BARRIERS TO IMPLEMENTATION OF EVIDENCE-BASED PRACTICE

Evidence–practice gaps evolve in two basic areas. One is related to EBP itself and the other is related to changing behavior.

Gaps may exist because of a lack of awareness of how to practice EBP or because of barriers to practicing it once these skills are developed. Numerous studies have addressed these barriers and consistently found that lack of awareness of how to search the literature, lack of critical appraisal skills, and, most importantly, lack of time are perceived barriers to practicing EBP.[24–31] This issue of *Hand Clinics* provides resources to assist with reducing many of these barriers.

However, knowing what to do, and doing it, are two different things. Implementing new evidence means changing behavior. Substantial evidence, particularly in psychologic, addiction, and health promotion research, indicates that it is not easy to change behavior, either on an individual or a group level. Making matters more complicated is the fact that clinicians work within the complex environments of different health care systems, clinics, and teams, which affects individual and group attitudes and behaviors regarding current clinical practice and any potential for change.

THEORETIC ASPECTS OF KNOWLEDGE TRANSLATION

All human actions have one or more of these seven causes: chance, nature, compulsion, habit, reason, passion, and desire.
  —Aristotle, Greek critic, philosopher, physicist, and zoologist (384 BC–322 BC)

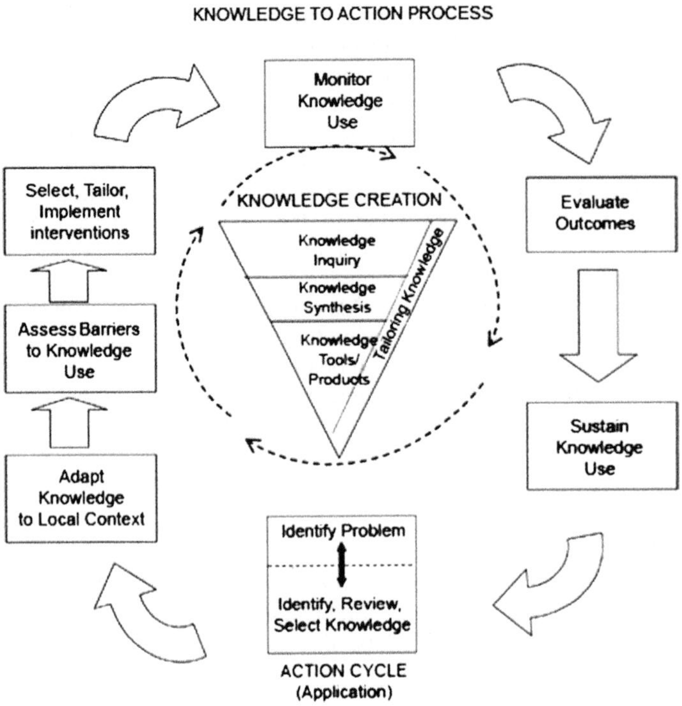

KNOWLEDGE TO ACTION PROCESS

Fig. 1. KTA process. (*From* Graham ID, Logan J, Harrison MB, et al. Lost in knowledge translation. J Contin Educ Health Prof 2006;26:13–24; with permission.)

Overview of Relevant Theoretic Frameworks

Theory or conceptual frameworks can be particularly important in an emerging field, particularly when the field draws on multiple disciplines, as in the case of KT. As yet, no single framework is accepted, nor do any completely describe the complex processes involved. However, the authors highlight some of the predominant ones to offer some foundation for the topic.

The theory of diffusion of innovation

The diffusion of innovation theory is perhaps the oldest and most consistently cited "knowledge translation theory," although it was developed in the 1950s to explain the spread of new ideas.[32] The theory relies on a sociologic perspective, where innovation is communicated "through particular channels, over time, among the members of the social system."[32] Under this theory, innovations pass through specific stages of decision/adoption: awareness/knowledge, interest/persuasion, evaluation/decision, trial/implementation, and adoption/confirmation. When implementing new EBP, it is important to consider at what stage of this process the individual context currently exists. This theory defines the important characteristics of an innovation:

Relative advantage (the degree to which it is better than the current accepted standard practice)

Compatibility (the extent to which it is consistent with existing values, past experiences, and needs)

Complexity (the difficulty in understanding and using the innovation; in hand surgery and therapy, this would translate into the "hands-on" technical difficulty in performing the new approach and in obtaining/using necessary devices)

Trialability (the extent to which the intervention can be experimented with on a limited basis)

Observability (the extent to which a visible result [eg, "improved outcome"] is achieved)

The theory also identifies different adopter categories, as shown in **Table 1**.

One of the benefits of this theory is that it provides a rationale and framework for needing multiple interventions to change practice behaviors. Clearly, individual hand surgeons and therapists would fall into different adopter categories and be at different stages in the process of adoption of evidence-based innovations.

Principles around the diffusion of innovation have been applied to various circumstances. Notably, Greenhalgh and colleagues[33] extended the concepts to health service organization, based on systematic review and conceptual models of sociology, psychology, economics, clinical epidemiology, marketing, political science, and

Table 1
Adopter categories

Category	Identified Characteristics
Innovators	Daring, risky, have sufficient control of financial resources to absorb possible loss, able to understand and apply complex technical knowledge, able to cope with uncertainty
Early adopters	Integrated in a social system, usually hold the greatest degree of opinion leadership, frequently serve as role models, respected by peers, successful
Early majority	Frequently interact with peers, seldom hold positions of opinion leadership, usually the largest component of the system, deliberate before adopting new ideas
Late majority	Usually one third of the system, react to pressure from peers, motivated by economic necessity, skeptical, cautious
Laggards	Not opinion leaders, usually more isolated, suspicious of innovation, tend to focus on the past, require long decision processes, may have limited resources

information/communication technology. They extracted four key characteristics of innovation within health care systems across these different disciplines and evaluated concepts around best practice. In so doing, they defined innovation and health service delivery as "a set of behaviors, routine, and ways of working along with any associated administrative technologies and systems which are 1. Perceived as new by a proportion of key stakeholders; 2. Linked to the provision or support of health care; 3. Discontinuous with previous practice; 4. Directed at improving health outcomes, administrative efficiency, cost effectiveness, or user experience; and 5. Implemented by means of planned and coordinated action by individuals, teams or organizations."

The theories of planned behavior

A theory that has risen to some predominance in KT work is the theory of planned behavior,[34,35] which suggests that individual behavior is driven by behavioral intentions. Behavioral intentions are a function of attitudes specifically about that behavior, the subjective norms (professional/cultural expectations) that relate to the performance of that behavior, and the individual's perception of his/her ability to perform or change the behavior. Differing from the diffusion of innovation theory, which is more a sociologic theory and focuses on the group, the theory of "planned behavior" is a social psychology theory focusing on the individual. This theoretic approach has proved useful in KT research and intervention planning because it directs areas that can be assessed and targeted to improve the use of best evidence. Research studies have shown that this model can explain, in part, changes in practice behavior

that occur with KT. Attitudes toward a clinical practice behavior (positive or negative) can be elicited qualitatively from interviews or focus groups. Their relative importance within target audiences can then be determined using surveys of the target audience, thus providing specific direction on areas that should be targeted for educational or other KT interventions.

The overall "attitude" is determined from the summed individual consequence and desirability assessments for all expected consequences of the behavior. The subjective norm is the individual's perception of whether "important" people (eg, professional colleagues or mentors) think the behavior should be performed. It is usually weighted by the motivation that an individual has to comply with the wishes of that person/body. Behavioral control is one's perception of the difficulty of performing a behavior. These assessments often consider how able the person is able to perform the action in the light of potential barriers. Practically speaking, it is perceived behavioral control that is measured, which may not be the same as actual control.

One of the valuable aspects of this theory is that it provides a framework to assess and plan for strategies on changing clinical practice. Information retrieved from the local context/players can identify specific components of the model and the nature of those influences, which can then be targeted for educational or other KT interventions. For example, if subjective norms are identified as an important element, opinion leaders may be indicated and the specific content of their messaging will be based on the evidence and the content of the subjective norms (**Fig. 2**).

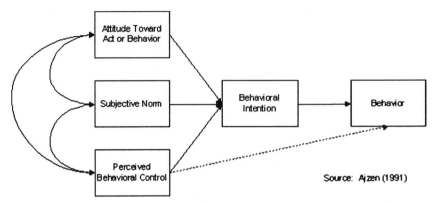

Fig. 2. The theory of planned behavior, which describes behavior as rising from intentions that are composed of the components illustrated. It is relevant to KT because changing behavior may require understanding and addressing people's attitudes about the behavior (positive and negative), their perceptions about what is considered the norm with their peers or profession, and the extent to which they feel they can change their behavior, given their environmental/personal situation. (*From* Ajzen I. From intentions to actions: a theory of planned behavior. Action-control: from cognition to behavior. Heidelberg, Germany: Springer; 1985. p. 11–39; with kind permission of Springer Science + Business Media.)

PRACTICAL ASPECTS OF KNOWLEDGE TRANSLATION

Everybody gets so much information all day long that they lose their common sense.
—Gertrude Stein, American author in France (1874–1946)

No theory fully explains the complex processes that govern how knowledge moves into action in clinical environments.[36] In fact, studies typically show that mathematic models based on these theories explain a small percentage of the variation in behavior.[37,38] So although conceptual frameworks or theories can provide guideposts on how to approach KT, a strong rationale remains to emphasize the importance of "common sense and experience."[36] For example, simple interventions like ensuring that proper equipment/supplies are readily available at the point of care might be sufficient to make great changes in use. Thus, KT is highly dependent on capturing the practical wisdom and engaging end users to define, customize, and implement the best decisions and to follow through to sustained action.

THE ACTION CYCLE: HOW TO APPROACH KNOWLEDGE TRANSLATION PROCESS

Take time to deliberate, but when the time for action has arrived, stop thinking and go in.
—Napoleon Bonaparte, French general and politician (1769–1821)

The process through which knowledge becomes actionable is, by nature, one that involves local contextualization, management, and ongoing support, which can be challenging for the surgeon or therapist and often requires a broader level of collaboration than is required for the management of individual patients. Various approaches have been suggested to provide structure to the KT process. A study conducted by Graham[39] of more than 60 different theories or frameworks identified some commonalities that provide guideposts for this process. The authors have adapted this list as follows, so it can be generalized to any practice:

- Identify the problem (aspect of practice) that needs to be addressed.
- Identify, review, and select the knowledge relevant to the problem that should be implemented.
- Adapt this knowledge to your local context (define the specific actions/practices that apply to your practice).
- Assess any potential barriers to the use of this knowledge (attitudinal, process, system, and so forth).
- Select, tailor, plan, and implement specific actions or KT interventions that are required to implement the change (see the description of some KT interventions below).
- Monitor knowledge use (define and monitor indicators that indicate whether the knowledge is being used [process]).
- Evaluate outcomes (define and monitor the outcome measures that reflect the impact of the targeted behavior [eg, patient outcomes]).

- Sustain ongoing knowledge use (plan for updating your practices as new knowledge arises).

The first stage of this process involves coming to a common understanding about the problem to which new evidence is to be applied. This early stage should not be bypassed because unless agreement exists as to which aspects of current clinical practice need to be changed, and which outcomes could be improved, it is unlikely that the rest of the process will be embraced. The next step has been well described through this text; EBP is the process of finding and evaluating the best clinical evidence to make clinical decisions. Until recently, less attention has been directed at how one might adapt this new knowledge to the local context. This stage requires selecting the relevant, effective, efficient, and feasible approaches that apply to a given clinical environment. This stage acknowledges that not all quality evidence can be implemented, nor is appropriate in every clinical situation. End users have the responsibility and burden of sifting through evidence-based recommendations and making decisions about what can, and should be, implemented.

The next stage involves assessment of potential barriers to the implementation of knowledge. Typically, interviews, questionnaires, and group discussions with different end users are used to identify potential barriers. Barriers may exist at various levels within individuals or systems. Some groups approach the assessment of barriers within a theoretic framework, whereas others adopt a more open-ended, qualitative approach, letting the participants reveal the barriers. Once potential barriers have been identified, their importance can be accessed on a larger scale through surveys or analysis of practice variation. For example, variations among different clinics/settings on guideline implementation may reveal organizational or process barriers and facilitators.

A KT strategy for any given individual or organization involves selection of specific "KT interventions" directed toward minimizing the local barriers or supporting implementation. Like clinical interventions, KT interventions have various indications and levels of effectiveness. Like clinical practice, KT practice has an element of science and an element of art. Although identification of barriers is always possible, ameliorating them does not necessarily result in changes in behavior. For example, numerous studies have identified that a lack of ability to search electronic databases is a perceived barrier to EBP.[24,26,40–42] However, workshops that train end users in searching have not been shown to increase the use of evidence or to affect patient outcomes.[43]

Methods of implementation should be open to creative solutions. In fact, brainstorming and creativity are essential to coming up with innovative, feasible, and potentially cost-effective solutions. For example, Ashe and colleagues[44] demonstrated that low-cost reminders called "wristwatch," where patients transferred letters to their family physicians and hand clinics faxed similar information, resulted in more than 90% improvement in investigation for osteoporosis following distal radius fracture. Wide engagement of stakeholders in the brainstorming process is more likely to facilitate innovative, action-oriented ideas. Experience suggests that restricting this process to clinicians is ill advised because most clinicians will readily suggest familiar interventions, like continuing education, which is minimally effective.

PROMOTING ACTION ON RESEARCH IMPLEMENTATION IN A HEALTH SERVICES FRAMEWORK

A framework entitled Promoting Action on Research Implementation in Health Services (PARIHS) was developed to represent the complexity of change processes involved in implementing EBP.[45,46] Successful research implementation is considered to be a function of the relationships among evidence, context, and facilitation (**Fig. 3**). Successful implementation is more likely if research evidence is clear and of high quality. However, the framework also emphasizes the importance of using clinical experience, patient experience, and local data/information as contributing evidence. In fact, where any of these pieces of information is seen as the only available evidence (isolation), action is compromised. Context is considered as a mediator of implementation. Contextual factors that promote successful implementation are categorized under the three broad themes of culture, leadership, and evaluation. "Learning" organizations that pay attention to individuals, group processes, and organizational systems are optimal. Transformative leadership and ongoing evaluation with feedback are important elements of context. The model acknowledges the importance of facilitation, where individuals carry out specific roles that aim to help others to change their clinical practice. Facilitation can be characterized by its purpose and role and the skills/attributes required of the facilitator.

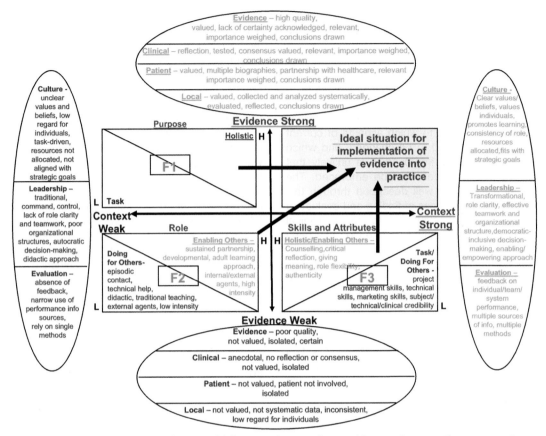

Fig. 3. The concepts in the PARIHS framework, illustrate the complexity of factors that contributes to moving evidence into practice within a system. Negative circumstances are in brown and positive in green. Context moves from negative (*left*) to positive (*right*) as the culture, leadership, and evaluation characteristics of the organization move toward facilitating positive change. Similarly, as the evidence (research, clinical, patient, and local) shifts from weak/isolated evidence to strong and comprehensive evidence, change is also facilitated. It is through mechanisms designed to facilitate adoption of new "best practices" that implementation can succeed. Characteristics of how change is facilitated through purpose, role and skills, and attributes can also provide weak or strong facilitation within environments. The balance of these factors creates the unique opportunity and challenges for adoption of EBP within different clinical settings.

The theory led to the development of a self-assessment (diagnostic/evaluative) tool that those implementing EBP can use to review and subsequently plan or evaluate strategies for implementation. This tool is available at http://www.ferasi.umontreal.ca/Pr%C3%A9sentations/PARiHS%20SAT%20A%20KITSON%2026%20OCT%2007.pdf.

KNOWLEDGE TRANSLATION INTERVENTIONS

Various specific KT interventions can be used to increase awareness of a problem, develop useable/actionable forms of evidence, inform end users about the evidence, and promote change in practice. Literature synthesis is one form of KT and is partially addressed in other articles in this issue (eg, systematic reviews). Thus, the authors highlight other KT interventions that are meant to promote change in clinical practice.

An important source of evidence on the effectiveness of KT interventions is the Effective Practice and Organization of Care (EPOC) group of the Cochrane Collaboration (http://www.epoc.cochrane.org/en/about.html). The EPOC group undertakes systematic reviews of interventions designed to improve professional practice and the delivery of effective health services, including various forms of continuing education, quality assurance, informatics, and financial, organizational, and regulatory interventions that can affect the ability of health care professionals to deliver services more effectively and efficiently (**Tables 2–12**).

Table 2
Printed material

Question	Answer
What is it?	Printed materials are written documents that summarize information or evidence.
What is the evidence?	They are most effective when combined with other educational efforts, such as toolkits, feedback, and communication between instructors and learners.[47,48]
When should it be used?	Printed materials are useful to reach a broad audience at low cost, particularly to increase awareness or provide resource/contact information for future reference; can be targeted for waiting areas or areas frequented by the target end user (eg, patient information brochures, drug marketing materials).
How should it be optimized?	Use clear language of an appropriate reading level and cultural presentation, visually appealing, relevant content.[49–52]

Data from Freemantle N, Harvey EL, Wolf F, et al. Printed educational materials: effects on professional practice and health care outcomes. Cochrane Database Syst Rev 2000;2:CD000172.

Table 3
Continuing education

Question	Answer
What is it?	CE is the most common structured information resource accessed by clinicians. It typically involves face-to-face workshops or, more recently, electronic and online learning. Various presentation styles, formats, pedagogic approaches, and structures have been used.
What is the evidence?	The validity of research into CE is limited by poor-quality evaluation methods.[53] Few studies have specifically addressed the attainment of surgical skills.[54] Controlled trials suggest that effectiveness is enhanced by personal feedback and work prompts. Qualitative studies have demonstrated that education plays only a small part in influencing doctors' behavior.[55] Traditional CE methods such as conferences have little direct impact on improving professional practice.[56–58] Active learning activities and interactive approaches are more effective than passive learning strategies.
When should it be used?	CE remains highly preferred by clinicians and can be useful across a broad array of contexts.
How should it be optimized?	Use active learning strategies (eg, knowledge pre- and posttests, audience engagement, hands-on activities, interactivity, multiple formats) and follow-up activities and evaluations. Emphasize relevant, practical, and current information that meets the needs of the end-user group.

Abbreviation: CE, continuing education.
Data from Refs.[59–61]

Table 4
Clinical practice guidelines

Question	Answer
What is it?	CPGs are systematically developed statements that provide specific information on the management of patients. In EBP, it is implied that these are formally developed using an evidence-based approach.[62]
What is the evidence?	Evidence indicates that clinicians who develop CPGs without adequate balance from expert methodologists are more likely to depart from evidence.[63,64] However, involvement of clinicians is also critical to relevance and acceptance. Evidence suggests that written guidelines without accompanying dissemination activities have little impact. Limited evidence suggests that they improve patient outcomes within specific contexts.[65] Changes in practice are more easily achieved with simple guidelines, like prescribing practices, as compared with more complex management issues. Current hand therapy practice guidelines appear to be of low quality.[66]
When should it be used?	CPGs can be used to make recommendations around the use of a specific intervention or on the comprehensive management of the specific problem. They require a sufficient body of quality evidence to make comprehensive recommendations and a multidisciplinary team committed to the development and dissemination of the end product.
How should it be optimized?	Engage multiple stakeholders including various disciplines, and experts in guideline development, patients, researchers, practicing clinicians, and professional associations. Use recognized methods for collection and synthesis of evidence and for achieving consensus.[67] Make recommendations clear, specific, and actionable. Provide supporting tools for implementation. See AGREE collaboration (http://www.agreecollaboration.org/) and The Guidelines International Network (http://www.g-i-n.net/). CPGs need to be kept up to date.

Abbreviations: AGREE, appraisal of guidelines, research, and evaluation; CPG, clinical practice guidelines.

Table 5
Audit and feedback

Question	Answer
What is it?	Audit and feedback is a process of monitoring that involves evaluating and providing feedback on clinical performance (against a defined acceptable standard); it can be verbal, electronic, or written.
What is the evidence?	Evidence is insufficient for accurate definition of the optimal approaches; however, a Cochrane review of 118 trials indicated that small-to-moderate changes in clinical practice can be expected (median 5%; range 16% to 70%). Contrary to expectations, audit and feedback is more useful where the behavior is less compatible with current norms.[52,68–70]
When should it be used?	Audit and feedback is applicable across various contexts; it requires definable standards that are explicit so that it is possible to define and evaluate adherence across most cases (eg, use of radiograph or outcome measures). It may be less useful for issues that are implicit, where decisions have to be customized to each patient (extent of repair, type of exercise). It should target where compliance is low and where perceived peer pressure is deemed a key determinant.
How should it be optimized?	Make informed decisions about the match between context and design of the audit and feedback in terms of content (comparative or not, anonymous or not; key message/behaviors; process and comparators); type (electronic, verbal, written); intensity (how often, how intrusive); method of delivery (post, peer, nonpeer, supervisor; reminders outreach visits); duration (how long); context (site). Make actions clear, based on strong evidence and compliance achievable in (nearly) all cases.

Data from Refs.[71–73]

Table 6
Educational outreach

Question	Answer
What is it?	Educational outreach is a personal visit by a trained person to health professionals in their own setting (also called academic detailing, educational detailing, public interest detailing).[74] It uses simple key messages, targeting of practitioners with low compliance, and delivery of the information by a respected person; it may be included with audit and feedback.
What is the evidence?	Small-to-moderate effects have been demonstrated, mostly for prescribing practices, with less evidence and variable effects in other areas of practice.[75]
When should it be used?	Educational outreach should be used when clear messages about changing specific clinical practices are possible.
How should it be optimized?	Use recognized experts who are financially independent from the industry or developer.

Table 7
Knowledge brokers

Question	Answer
What is it?	Knowledge brokers enable the linking of decision makers with researchers, facilitating their interaction to allow each to better understand the goals, cultures, and environmental limitations of each other's work, and allowing them to work collaboratively on the use of evidence for decision making.[76–79]
What is the evidence?	Knowledge brokers have been less studied than other KT interventions.
When should it be used?	They should be used where changes in policy are needed and where common goals/outcomes can be achieved among policy makers, end users, and knowledge developers.
How should it be optimized?	Trust and development of common ground are essential. See case examples and supports available from the Canadian Health Services Research Foundation (http://www.chsrf.ca/brokering/index_e.php).

Table 8
Opinion leaders

Question	Answer
What is it?	OLs (innovative, socially connected, and respected persons) are used to champion a behavior directly or indirectly (through attitudes). In medicine, key OLs are perceived by others to be influential (typically recognized as belonging to a specific area of expertise or specialty). It is uncertain whether the expertise or specialty is the defining characteristic of OLs; it appears more that others see them as being knowledgeable, credible, influential.
What is the evidence?	An overall improvement of 10%[80] in behavior has been reported.
When should it be used?	OLs should be used when changes in attitude are critical to obtaining practice change, where the end users or their specific behaviors are difficult to identify, and in professions or areas of practice where it has been identified that social norms are an important component of decision making or if specific interventions are associated with OLs.
How should it be optimized?	Accurately identify the OLs for the specific behavior or intervention (not generic).

Abbreviation: OL, opinion leader.

Table 9
Incentives

Question	Answer
What is it?	Incentives means provision of rewards (often monetary) for performance of specific actions or achieving specific outcomes. One specific form of incentive is pay for performance, an emerging movement in health insurance where providers are awarded for meeting specific targets when providing health care.
What is the evidence?	A systematic review of the impact of industry funding on the outcomes of clinical research studies has indicated that in several areas, including pharmaceutic,[81,82] spinal,[83] and orthopedic surgery research,[84] the presence of industry funding is associated with an increased likelihood of finding a positive advantage for the funder's product. Another review concluded that "Financial relationships among industry, scientific investigators, and academic institutions are widespread. Conflicts of interest arising from these ties can influence biomedical research in important ways."[85] These financial incentives have the potential to "contaminate" EBP. A systematic review of empiric studies of the relationship between financial incentives designed to improve health care and a quantitative measure of health quality identified 17 different studies with various levels of incentive (individual physician, provider group, or health care payment system). Most (13/17) studies evaluated the process of care, not patient outcomes. Five of the 6 studies addressing physician-level financial incentives and 7 of the 9 studies for provider group–level incentives found positive effects on measures of quality. One of the 2 studies of incentives at the payment system level found a positive effect on access to care and 1 showed evidence of a negative effect for the sickest patients. Four studies indicated that unintended consequences arose. The evidence is not clear on either effectiveness or indications for the optimal situation when incentives should be enacted. Sustainability is variable; compliance may drop off when incentives decrease.
When should it be used?	Preliminary evidence and health care policy/ethics suggest that incentive programs must be designed so as not to disadvantage those who have more complex or difficult problems.
How should it be optimized?	Incorporate patient and process outcomes in ongoing monitoring of the impact of the incentives; ensure adequate compensation for both simple and complicated cases; initiate processes to monitor and deal with unintended consequences.

Table 10
Regulation

Question	Answer
What is it?	A regulation is a public policy or professional licensure policy that mandates compliance with specific behaviors/practices.
What is the evidence?	Evidence is limited and difficult to determine because few studies have specifically focused on the role of regulation and it can be difficult to assess behavior change accurately once regulations are in place.
When should it be used?	Regulations should be used when voluntary compliance has failed, and in areas where clear evidence exists about specific actions that should be taken. It is easier to enact for simple behaviors like prescribing practices/implant selection (eg, FDA) or access to care.
How should it be optimized?	Involve opinion leaders and professional associations in the development/definition and dissemination of the new policy or regulation. Lead-in time should have a phase where voluntary compliance or audit and feedback is incorporated. Implement clear policy recommendations and identify a clear rationale for changes in policy.

Abbreviation: FDA, Food and Drug Administration.

Table 11
Decision aids

Question	Answer
What is it?	Decision aids are tools developed to assist patients or practitioners to make specific decisions using available evidence where it is important to weigh potential benefits and risks, or different options and their potential outcomes. See a one-page pdf fillable example (http://decisionaid.ohri.ca/docs/das/OPDG.pdf) that can be used across generic decisions or a two-page hard copy version (http://decisionaid.ohri.ca/docs/das/OPDG_2pg.pdf) of the Ottawa decision guide as an example.
What is the evidence?	Orthopedic surgeons have a positive attitude about the use of patient decision aids in joint replacement surgery.[86] However, physicians' intentions to use decision aids are often not consistent with practice behaviors.[39] A systematic review indicated that patient decision aids improve decision quality and the perception of being informed or understanding values; however, the size of the effect varies across studies.[87,88]
When should it be used?	Decision aids should be used when one or more reasonable investigational or treatment options exist with varying types of effects or risks for complication (eg, implant surgery).
How should it be optimized?	Use a guide to assist with development of a patient decision aid (http://decisionaid.ohri.ca/) or search for decision aids that are already developed; an online tutorial is also available (https://decisionaid.ohri.ca/ODST/). The Cochrane Library also provides a decision aid library (https://decisionaid.ohri.ca/DALI/). Follow quality criteria.[89]

Table 12
Clinical decision rules

Question	Answer
What is it?	Clinical decision rules are a specific kind of decision aid for clinicians, containing variables from the history, physical examination, or simple diagnostic tests that are used in combination to make a decision (ie, diagnose, determine the need for a specific test, or implement a specific treatment action).
What is the evidence?	Studies suggest that the use of well-developed clinical decision rules results in less radiography and less time spent in the emergency department, and does not decrease patient satisfaction or result in misdiagnosis.[90]
When should it be used?	Clinical decision rules are particularly useful for combining clinical tests, imaging, or other diagnostic tests into an overall diagnosis where sufficient evidence on the value of the individual diagnostic features allows for a rigorous and well-grounded cohort study to be conducted determining the optimal combination and weighting of the components to make the best diagnosis/clinical decision. Also useful for making decisions about ordering additional tests, particularly imaging, the classic example being the Ottawa ankle rules.[91–93]
How should it be optimized?	Use rigorous methodology to develop[94–97] and involve stakeholder in setting the priority for an implementation of the clinical decision rules.

KEY MESSAGES

Knowledge, if it does not determine action, is dead to us.
    —Plotinus, Roman philosopher (205 AD– 270 AD)

The key messages of this article may be summarized as follows. Additional tools are available in **Appendix 1**.

1. The benefits of EBP depend on KT, moving evidence into practice.
2. KT should be embedded in the creation of knowledge and drive new knowledge inquiry.
3. KT should consider and apply theory that informs our understanding of how systems and individuals change and use knowledge.
4. KT must capture the embedded practical knowledge on barriers and solutions that exist within systems and end users.
5. New knowledge must be customized to meet the needs of different end users and transformed into useable formats.
6. The effectiveness of different isolated KT interventions varies; combined interventions are often more effective, particularly in complex situations with diverse end users (or when addressing different barriers).
7. Passive educational interventions, including professional education conferences and written guidelines, are unlikely to change professional behavior, if used alone.
8. More recent KT interventions, like evidence-based clinical practice guidelines, clinical decision rules, patient decision aids, audit and feedback, pay for performance, opinion leaders, and knowledge brokering, are potentially beneficial but have not yet been evaluated specifically in hand surgery or hand therapy practices.
9. Providing the right information, in the right format, at the right time is important.

APPENDIX 1
Useful Knowledge Translation Web Sites/Tools

KT+   (http://plus.mcmaster.ca/KT/Default. aspx). This alerting service provides the current evidence on "T2" KT (ie, research addressing the knowledge to practice gap), including published original articles and systematic reviews on health care quality improvement, continuing professional education, computerized clinical decision support, health services research, and patient adherence. Its purpose is to inform those working in the KT area of current research as it is published.

The Canadian Health Services Research Foundation (http://www.chsrf.ca/home_e. php). This foundation supports the evidence-informed management of Canada's health care system by facilitating knowledge transfer and exchange, bridging the gap between research and health care management and policy.

KT Clearinghouse (http://knowledgetranslation. ca/ktclearinghouse/home) This clearinghouse provides information, resources, and tools for KT.

Knowledge Translation Program, Faculty of Medicine, University of Toronto. (http://www.ktp.utoronto.ca/).

National Center for the Dissemination of Disability Research Disability (http://www.ncddr.org/). The center's scope of work focuses on KT of National Institute on Disability and Rehabilitative Research-sponsored research and development results into evidence-based instruments and systematic reviews. NCDDR is developing systems for applying rigorous standards of evidence in describing, assessing, and disseminating research and development outcomes.

The Canadian Institutes of Health Research (http://www.cihr-irsc.gc.ca/e/29418.html). The Canadian (national) research funding agency has a strong focus on KT.

REFERENCES

1. Alderman AK, Chung KC, Demonner S, et al. The rheumatoid hand: a predictable disease with unpredictable surgical practice patterns. Arthritis Rheum 2002;47(5):537–42.
2. Alderman AK, Arora AS, Kuhn L, et al. An analysis of women's and men's surgical priorities and willingness to have rheumatoid hand surgery. J Hand Surg [Am] 2006;31(9):1447–53.
3. Alderman AK, Ubel PA, Kim HM, et al. Surgical management of the rheumatoid hand: consensus and controversy among rheumatologists and hand surgeons. J Rheumatol 2003;30(7):1464–72.
4. Alderman AK, Chung KC, Kim HM, et al. Effectiveness of rheumatoid hand surgery: contrasting perceptions of hand surgeons and rheumatologists. J Hand Surg [Am] 2003;28(1):3–11.
5. Pettersson K, Wagnsjo P, Hulin E. NeuFlex compared with Sutter prostheses: a blind, prospective, randomised comparison of silastic metacarpophalangeal joint prostheses. Scand J Plast Reconstr Surg Hand Surg 2006;40(5):284–90.
6. Parkkila TJ, Belt EA, Hakala M, et al. Grading of radiographic osteolytic changes after silastic

metacarpophalangeal arthroplasty and a prospective trial of osteolysis following use of Swanson and Sutter prostheses. J Hand Surg [Br] 2005;30(4):382–7.
7. Moller K, Sollerman C, Geijer M, et al. Avanta versus Swanson silicone implants in the MCP joint–a prospective, randomized comparison of 30 patients followed for 2 years. J Hand Surg [Br] 2005;30(1):8–13.
8. Delaney R, Trail IA, Nuttall D. A comparative study of outcome between the Neuflex and Swanson metacarpophalangeal joint replacements. J Hand Surg [Br] 2005;30(1):3–7.
9. McArthur PA, Milner RH. A prospective randomized comparison of Sutter and Swanson silastic spacers. J Hand Surg [Br] 1998;23(5):574–7.
10. Schmidt K, Witt K, Ossowski A, et al [Therapy of rheumatoid destruction of the middle finger metacarpophalangeal joint with a Swanson silastic implant stabilized resection arthroplasty: comparative study of long and intermediate term results with and without implantation of titanium grommets]. Z Rheumatol 1997;56(5):287–97 [German].
11. Sollerman CJ, Geijer M. Polyurethane versus silicone for endoprosthetic replacement of the metacarpophalangeal joints in rheumatoid arthritis. Scand J Plast Reconstr Surg Hand Surg 1996;30(2):145–50.
12. Pereira JA, Belcher HJ. A comparison of metacarpophalangeal joint silastic arthroplasty with or without crossed intrinsic transfer. J Hand Surg [Br] 2001;26(3):229–34.
13. Ring D, Simmons BP, Hayes M. Continuous passive motion following metacarpophalangeal joint arthroplasty. J Hand Surg [Am] 1998;23(3):505–11.
14. Healy C, Mulhall KJ, Bouchier-Hayes DJ, et al. Practice patterns in flexor tendon repair. Ir J Med Sci 2007;176(1):41–4.
15. MacDermid JC, Roth JH, McMurty R. Predictors of time lost from work following a distal radius fracture. J Occup Rehabil 2007;17(1):47–62.
16. Michlovitz SL, LaStayo PC, Alzner S, et al. Distal radius fractures: therapy practice patterns. J Hand Ther 2001;14(4):249–57.
17. Trudel D, Duley J, Zastrow I, et al. Rehabilitation for patients with lateral epicondylitis: a systematic review. J Hand Ther 2004;17(2):243–66.
18. Schuster MA, McGlynn EA, Brook RH. How good is the quality of health care in the United States? Milbank Q 1998;76(4):517–63 509.
19. Mangione-Smith R, DeCristofaro AH, Setodji CM, et al. The quality of ambulatory care delivered to children in the United States. N Engl J Med 2007;357(15):1515–23.
20. Asch SM, Kerr EA, Keesey J, et al. Who is at greatest risk for receiving poor-quality health care? N Engl J Med 2006;354(11):1147–56.

21. Estabrooks CA. Mapping the research utilization field in nursing. Can J Nurs Res 1999;31(1):53–72.
22. Estabrooks CA. Translating research into practice: implications for organizations and administrators. Can J Nurs Res 2003;35(3):53–68.
23. Estabrooks CA, Thompson DS, Lovely JJ, et al. A guide to knowledge translation theory. J Contin Educ Health Prof 2006;26(1):25–36.
24. Bennett S, Tooth L, McKenna K, et al. Perceptions of evidence-based practice: a survey of Australian occupational therapists. Aust Occ Ther J 2003; 50(1):13–22.
25. Bialocerkowski AE, Grimmer KA, Milanese SF, et al. Application of current research evidence to clinical physiotherapy practice. J Allied Health 2004;33(4): 230–7.
26. Dysart AM, Tomlin GS. Factors related to evidence-based practice among U.S. occupational therapy clinicians. Am J Occup Ther 2002;56(3):275–84.
27. Kamwendo K. What do Swedish physiotherapists feel about research? A survey of perceptions, attitudes, intentions and engagement. Physiother Res Int 2002;7(1):23–34.
28. Maher CG, Sherrington C, Elkins M, et al. Challenges for evidence-based physical therapy: accessing and interpreting high-quality evidence on therapy. Phys Ther 2004;84(7):644–54.
29. McCluskey A. Occupational therapists report on low level of knowledge, skill and involvement in evidence-based practice. Aust Occ Ther J 2003; 50(1):3–12.
30. Palfreyman S, Tod A, Doyle J. Comparing evidence-based practice of nurses and physiotherapists. Br J Nurs 2003;12(4):246–53.
31. Young JM, Ward JE. Evidence-based medicine in general practice: beliefs and barriers among Australian GPs. J Eval Clin Pract 2001;7(2):201–10.
32. Rogers EM. Diffusion of innovation. New York: The Free Press; 1962. Ref Type: Report.
33. Greenhalgh T, Glenn R, Macfarlane F, et al. Diffusion of innovations in health service organisations: a systematic literature review. London: Blackwell BMJ Books; 2005.
34. Ajzen I. From intentions to actions: a theory of planned behavior. Action-control: from cognition to behavior. Heidelberg (Germany): Springer; 1985. p. 11–39.
35. Ajzen I. The theory of planned behavior. Organ Behav Hum Decis Process 1991;50:179–211.
36. Bhattacharyya O, Reeves S, Garfinkel S, et al. Designing theoretically-informed implementation interventions: fine in theory, but evidence of effectiveness in practice is needed. Implement Sci 2006;1:5.
37. Bonetti D, Pitts NB, Eccles M, et al. Applying psychological theory to evidence-based clinical practice: identifying factors predictive of taking intra-oral radiographs. Soc Sci Med 2006;63(7): 1889–99.
38. Godin G, Belanger-Gravel A, Eccles M, et al. Health-care professionals' intentions and behaviours: a systematic review of studies based on social cognitive theories. Implement Sci 2008;3:36.
39. Graham ID, Tetroe J. Some theoretical underpinnings of knowledge translation. Acad Emerg Med 2007;14(11):936–41.
40. Dubouloz CJ, Egan M, Vallerand J, et al. Occupational therapists' perceptions of evidence-based practice. Am J Occup Ther 1999;53(5):445–53.
41. Jette DU, Bacon K, Batty C, et al. Evidence-based practice: beliefs, attitudes, knowledge, and behaviors of physical therapists. Phys Ther 2003;83(9): 786–805.
42. Newman M, Papadopoulos I, Sigsworth J. Barriers to evidence-based practice. Intensive Crit Care Nurs 1998;14(5):231–8.
43. Coomarasamy A, Taylor R, Khan KS. A systematic review of postgraduate teaching in evidence-based medicine and critical appraisal. Med Teach 2003; 25(1):77–81.
44. Ashe M, Khan K, Guy P, et al. Wristwatch-distal radial fracture as a marker for osteoporosis investigation: a controlled trial of patient education and a physician alerting system. J Hand Ther 2004; 17(3):324–8.
45. Kitson A, Harvey G, McCormack B. Enabling the implementation of evidence based practice: a conceptual framework. Qual Health Care 1998;7(3):149–58.
46. Freemantle N, Harvey EL, Wolf F, et al. Printed educational materials: effects on professional practice and health care outcomes. Cochrane Database Syst Rev 2000;(2):CD000172.
47. Wong SS, Wilczynski NL, Haynes RB. Comparison of top-performing search strategies for detecting clinically sound treatment studies and systematic reviews in MEDLINE and EMBASE. J Med Libr Assoc 2006;94(4):451–5.
48. Farmer AP, Legare F, Turcot L, et al. Printed educational materials: effects on professional practice and health care outcomes. Cochrane Database Syst Rev 2008;(3):CD004398.
49. Paul CL, Redman S, Sanson-Fisher RW. A cost-effective approach to the development of printed materials: a randomized controlled trial of three strategies. Health Educ Res 2004;19(6):698–706.
50. Ekstrom I. Printed materials for an aging population: design considerations. J Biocommun 1993;20(3): 25–30.
51. Estey A, Jeremy P, Jones M. Developing printed materials for patients with visual deficiencies. J Ophthalmic Nurs Technol 1990;9(6):247–9.
52. Lange JW. Developing printed materials for patient education. Dimens Crit Care Nurs 1989;8(4):250–8.

53. Ratanawongsa N, Thomas PA, Marinopoulos SS, et al. The reported validity and reliability of methods for evaluating continuing medical education: a systematic review. Acad Med 2008;83(3):274–83.

54. Rogers DA, Elstein AS, Bordage G. Improving continuing medical education for surgical techniques: applying the lessons learned in the first decade of minimal access surgery. Ann Surg 2001;233(2):159–66.

55. Smith F, Singleton A, Hilton S. General practitioners' continuing education: a review of policies, strategies and effectiveness, and their implications for the future. Br J Gen Pract 1998;48(435):1689–95.

56. Davis DA, Thomson MA, Oxman AD, et al. Changing physician performance. A systematic review of the effect of continuing medical education strategies. JAMA 1995;274(9):700–5.

57. Eccles MP, Grimshaw JM. Selecting, presenting and delivering clinical guidelines: are there any "magic bullets"? Med J Aust 2004;180(Suppl 6):S52–4.

58. Grimshaw J, Freemantle N, Wallace S, et al. Developing and implementing clinical practice guidelines. Qual Health Care 1995;4(1):55–64.

59. Beggs C, Sumison T. After the workshop: a model to evaluate the long-term benefits of continuing education. Physiother Can 2004;49:279–91.

60. Davis D. Continuing education, guideline implementation, and the emerging transdisciplinary field of knowledge translation. J Contin Educ Health Prof 2006;26(1):5–12.

61. Davis D, O'Brien MA, Freemantle N, et al. Impact of formal continuing medical education: do conferences, workshops, rounds, and other traditional continuing education activities change physician behavior or health care outcomes? JAMA 1999;282(9):867–74.

62. Clinical practice guidelines: directions for a new program. Committee to Advise the Public Health on Clinical Practice Guidelines, Institute of Medicine. Washington (DC): National Academy Press; 1990.

63. Savoie I, Kazanjian A, Bassett K. Do clinical practice guidelines reflect research evidence? J Health Serv Res Policy 2000;5(2):76–82.

64. van der Sanden WJ, Mettes DG, Plasschaert AJ, et al. Development of clinical practice guidelines: evaluation of 2 methods. J Can Dent Assoc 2004;70(5):301.

65. Bahtsevani C, Uden G, Willman A. Outcomes of evidence-based clinical practice guidelines: a systematic review. Int J Technol Assess Health Care 2004;20(4):427–33.

66. MacDermid JC. The quality of clinical practice guidelines in hand therapy. J Hand Ther 2004;17(2):200–9.

67. Woolf SH, DiGuiseppi CG, Atkins D, et al. Developing evidence-based clinical practice guidelines: lessons learned by the US Preventive Services Task Force. Annu Rev Public Health 1996;17:511–38.

68. O'Brien MA, Oxman AD, Davis DA, et al. Audit and feedback versus alternative strategies: effects on professional practice and health care outcomes. Cochrane Database Syst Rev 1998;(1):CD000260.

69. Jamtvedt G, Young JM, Kristoffersen DT, et al. Does telling people what they have been doing change what they do? A systematic review of the effects of audit and feedback. Qual Saf Health Care 2006;15(6):433–6.

70. Jamtvedt G, Young JM, Kristoffersen DT, et al. Audit and feedback: effects on professional practice and health care outcomes. Cochrane Database Syst Rev 2006;(2):CD000259.

71. Foy R, MacLennan G, Grimshaw J, et al. Attributes of clinical recommendations that influence change in practice following audit and feedback. J Clin Epidemiol 2002;55(7):717–22.

72. Foy R, Eccles MP, Jamtvedt G, et al. What do we know about how to do audit and feedback? Pitfalls in applying evidence from a systematic review. BMC Health Serv Res 2005;5:50.

73. Thomson O'Brien MA, Oxman AD, Davis DA, et al. Audit and feedback versus alternative strategies: effects on professional practice and health care outcomes. Cochrane Database Syst Rev 2000;(2):CD000260.

74. Soumerai SB, Avorn J. Principles of educational outreach ('academic detailing') to improve clinical decision making. JAMA 1990;263(4):549–56.

75. O'Brien MA, Rogers S, Jamtvedt G, et al. Educational outreach visits: effects on professional practice and health care outcomes. Cochrane Database Syst Rev 2007;(4):CD000409.

76. Lomas J. The in-between world of knowledge brokering. BMJ 2007;334(7585):129–32.

77. van Kammen J, Jansen CW, Bonsel GJ, et al. Technology assessment and knowledge brokering: the case of assisted reproduction in The Netherlands. Int J Technol Assess Health Care 2006;22(3):302–6.

78. van Kammen J, de Savigny D, Sewankambo N. Using knowledge brokering to promote evidence-based policy-making: the need for support structures. Bull World Health Organ 2006;84(8):608–12.

79. Thomson O'Brien MA, Oxman AD, Haynes RB, et al. Local opinion leaders: effects on professional practice and health care outcomes. Cochrane Database Syst Rev 2000;(2):CD000125.

80. Doumit G, Gattellari M, Grimshaw J, et al. Local opinion leaders: effects on professional practice and health care outcomes. Cochrane Database Syst Rev 2007;(1):CD000125.

81. Jorgensen AW, Hilden J, Gotzsche PC. Cochrane reviews compared with industry supported meta-analyses and other meta-analyses of the same drugs: systematic review. BMJ 2006;333(7572):782.

82. Lexchin J, Bero LA, Djulbegovic B, et al. Pharmaceutical industry sponsorship and research

outcome and quality: systematic review. BMJ 2003; 326(7400):1167–70.

83. Shah RV, Albert TJ, Bruegel-Sanchez V, et al. Industry support and correlation to study outcome for papers published in Spine. Spine 2005;30(9):1099–104.

84. Leopold SS, Warme WJ, Fritz BE, et al. Association between funding source and study outcome in orthopaedic research. Clin Orthop Relat Res 2003;(415):293–301.

85. Bekelman JE, Li Y, Gross CP. Scope and impact of financial conflicts of interest in biomedical research: a systematic review. JAMA 2003;289(4):454–65.

86. Adam JA, Khaw FM, Thomson RG, et al. Patient decision aids in joint replacement surgery: a literature review and an opinion survey of consultant orthopaedic surgeons. Ann R Coll Surg Engl 2008; 90(3):198–207.

87. O'connor AM, Bennett C, Stacey D, et al. Do patient decision aids meet effectiveness criteria of the international patient decision aid standards collaboration? A systematic review and meta-analysis. Med Decis Making 2007;27(5):554–74.

88. O'connor AM, Drake ER, Fiset V, et al. The Ottawa patient decision aids. Eff Clin Pract 1999;2(4): 163–70.

89. Elwyn G, O'Connor A, Stacey D, et al. Developing a quality criteria framework for patient decision aids: online international Delphi consensus process. BMJ 2006;333(7565):417.

90. Perry JJ, Stiell IG. Impact of clinical decision rules on clinical care of traumatic injuries to the foot and ankle, knee, cervical spine, and head. Injury 2006; 37(12):1157–65.

91. Keogh SP, Shafi A, Wijetunge DB. Comparison of Ottawa ankle rules and current local guidelines for use of radiography in acute ankle injuries. J R Coll Surg Edinb 1998;43(5):341–3.

92. Leddy JJ, Smolinski RJ, Lawrence J, et al. Prospective evaluation of the Ottawa ankle rules in a university sports medicine center. With a modification to increase specificity for identifying malleolar fractures. Am J Sports Med 1998;26(2):158–65.

93. Mann CJ, Grant I, Guly H, et al. Use of the Ottawa ankle rules by nurse practitioners. J Accid Emerg Med 1998;15(5):315–6.

94. Shapiro SE. Guidelines for developing and testing clinical decision rules. West J Nurs Res 2006; 28(2):244–53.

95. Shapiro SE. Evaluating clinical decision rules. West J Nurs Res 2005;27(5):655–64.

96. McGinn TG, Guyatt GH, Wyer PC, et al. Guides to the medical literature: XXII: how to use articles about clinical decision rules. Evidence-Based Medicine Working Group. JAMA 2000;284(1):79–84.

97. Stiell IG, Wells GA. Methodologic standards for the development of clinical decision rules in emergency medicine. Ann Emerg Med 1999;33(4): 437–47.

Erratum

Nerve Transfers in Brachial Plexus Birth Palsies: Indications, Techniques, and Outcomes

Scott H. Kozin, MD[a,b],*

In the November 2008 issue "Nerve Transfers," in the article identified above, Figs. 3–25 and 27 were credited incorrectly. These images are courtesy of Shriners Hospital for Children. We apologize for this oversight.

[a] Department of Orthopaedic Surgery, Temple University, 3401 Broad Street, Philadelphia, PA 19140, USA
[b] Upper Extremity Center of Excellence, Shriner's Hospitals for Children, 3551 North Broad Street, Philadelphia, PA 19140, USA
* Upper Extremity Center of Excellence, Shriners Hospitals for Children, 3551 North Broad Street, Philadelphia, PA 19140.

Hand Clin 25 (2009) 145
doi:10.1016/j.hcl.2008.12.005

Index

Note: Page numbers of article titles are in **boldface** type.

A

American College of Physicians Journal Club Plus, 19–20, 21
Arthroscopic repairs, and mini-open repairs, of rotator cuff, equivalency between, support by evidence?, **67–70**
Australian/Canadian Hand Osteoarthritis Index (AusCan Index), 98, 100

B

Biomedical clinician-centered approach to illness, 86
Biopsyhosocial approach, patient-centered evidence-based, to illness, 86–87
British Medical Journal, BMJ Clinical Evidence, 22–23

C

Canadian Occupational Performance Measure (COPM), 98, 100
Carpal tunnel release, economic evaluation of, 116
Clinical practice, outcomes in, using evidence-based approach to measure, **97–111**
    problems associated with, 97–98
Clinician-centered approach, biomedical, to illness, 86
Cochrane Library database, 20, 22, 115
Communication skills, for shared decision-making in evidence-based medicine, 91–93
Consensus, diagnosis, and diagnostic criteria, **43–48**
    measurement of, 46
Critical appraisal/recommendations tools, online, 39–40
Cumulative Index to Nursing and Allied Health Literature (CINAHL), 20, 21

D

Decision-making, medical, models of, health provider-as-agent model, 84
    informed decision-making model, 84
    paternalistic model, 83–84
    patient-centered care, 85
    shared-decision model, 84–85
Diagnosis, as probabilistic concept, 47
    diagnostic criteria, and consensus, **43–48**
Diagnostic criteria, diagnosis, and consensus, **43–48**
    reliable, need for, 47
Diagnostic scale(s), creation of, 44–45

gold standards, 45–46
reporting of results of, 46–47
Diagnostic tests, articles about, worksheet for evaluating and using, 13–16
    evaluation of quality of, 38
    evidence-based practice to select, **49–57**

E

Economic analysis, of new techniques, hand surgeons and, 113
Economic evaluation(s), characteristics of, 114
    consideration of relevant viewpoints in, 116–117
    in surgery of hand, **113–123**
    results of, validity of, 115–116
Evaluation form, for critical appraisal of study design for psychometric articles, 10
Evidence, moved into action, for accomplishment of health benefits, 125–126
    practice gap, as barrier to implementation of evidence-based practice, 127
    in hand surgery and therapy, 126–127
    evolution of, 127
Evidence-based approach, to measure outcomes in clinical practice, **97–111**
    problems associated with, 97–98
Evidence-based medicine, and treatment related to experience, 88
    electronic alert services for, 23, 24
    emotive power of words and, 87
    evidence retrieval for, future of, 24–25
    function of mind and effect on illness behavior, 88
    incomplete correlation between findings and words and, 87
    issues raised by, 87–88
    literature search at point of care, 22–23, 24
    practical examples of, 23–24
    "push out services" for, 23, 24
    resources for personal digital assistants, 24
    searching in, evidence-based medicine filters for, 18, 19
Evidence-based practice, adopter characteristics and, 129
    and literature search, 16–17
    and shared decision-making, communication skills for, 91–93
    optimizing communication in, 88–93
    application to patient, 33–41
    appraisal of evidence for validity and usefulness, 52–56

Hand Clin 25 (2009) 147–150
doi:10.1016/S0749-0712(08)00119-4

hand.theclinics.com

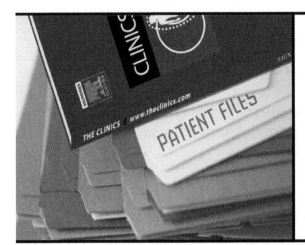
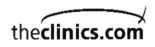

Moving?

Make sure your subscription moves with you!

To notify us of your new address, find your **Clinics Account Number** (located on your mailing label above your name), and contact customer service at:

E-mail: elspcs@elsevier.com

800-654-2452 (subscribers in the U.S. & Canada)
314-453-7041 (subscribers outside of the U.S. & Canada)

Fax number: 314-523-5170

Elsevier Periodicals Customer Service
11830 Westline Industrial Drive
St. Louis, MO 63146

*To ensure uninterrupted delivery of your subscription, please notify us at least 4 weeks in advance of move.

Printed and bound by CPI Group (UK) Ltd, Croydon, CR0 4YY

03/10/2024

01040352-0018